The process of change

The International Library of
Group Psychotherapy and Group Process

Therapeutic Communities Section

Section Editors

R.D. Hinshelwood
Consultant Psychotherapist
St Bernard's Hospital, Southall, Middlesex

Nick Manning
Lecturer in Social Policy and Administration
University of Kent

The process of change

Maxwell Jones
Consultant in Social Ecology and Psychiatry

Routledge & Kegan Paul
Boston, London, Melbourne and Henley

To Jimmy Millar and Cathy Wilson, my colleagues at Dingleton
Hospital, who made this project possible

First published in 1982
by Routledge & Kegan Paul Ltd
9 Park Street, Boston 02108, USA,
39 Store Street, London WC1E 7DD,
296 Beaconsfield Parade, Middle Park,
Melbourne, 3206, Australia and
Broadway House, Newtown Road,
Henley-on-Thames, Oxon RG9 1EN
Printed in Great Britain by
Billing & Son Ltd., Guildford and Worcester
Copyright © Maxwell Jones 1982

Library of Congress Cataloging in Publication Data

Jones, Maxwell.
The process of change.
Bibliography: P.
Includes index.
1. Therapeutic community - Case studies.
2. Learning - Social aspects - Case studies.
3. Social change - Case studies. I. Title.
RC489.T67J67   362.2'1   82-3874

ISBN 0-7100-9255-5   AACR2

Contents

Preface

During seven years as Physician Superintendent of Dingleton
Hospital in Melrose, Scotland, the process of change from a closed
to an open system was accomplished in collaboration with staff,
patients and the outside community. There are few, if any,
detailed descriptions of social systems in the process of change
over a period of years. I believe that this account is relevant to
all social systems in demonstrating that an open system is an ideal
setting for social learning, growth and creativity. It represents
one possible alternative as part of a counterculture to offset the
failure of Western society to achieve a stable and harmonious
world. The values of power, money and greed implicit in hierarchi
cal and bureaucratic systems can be replaced by an effective
communication network of information-sharing, shared decision-
making, social learning and growth.

Acknowledgments

I want to remember with gratitude those friends who acted as an inspiration for my early growth. Post-war Britain produced a remarkable group of Medical Superintendents who had a profound effect on the beginning of social psychiatry: Cecil Beaton of Portsmouth, T.P. Rees of Warlingham, Duncan McMillan of Nottingham, Rudolf Freudenberg of Netherne, David Clark of Fulbourn, Denis Martin of Claybury, Walter Maclay of Mill Hill, and my colleagues Ben Pomyrn, Bob Rapoport, Fergus Stallard, Joy Tuxford and Eileen Skellern at Henderson. In early post-war Europe A. Querido of the Amsterdam experiment; Peter Baan, creator of the Van der Hoven Clinic in Utrecht; Herluf Thomstad in Oslo; P. Sivadon in Paris; A. Repond in the canton of Valais in Switzerland; Bengt Berggren of Stockholm; and in North America Paul Polak, Ernie Gruenberg of Columbia University in New York, John Cumming in Saskatchewan, Al Kraft at Fort Logan in Denver, Dennie Briggs and Doug Grant in California.

Introduction

Learning as a social process, growth and creativity form the main focus of this story of Dingleton Hospital. What began as a therapeutic community in a mental hospital came to involve wider parameters in schools, prisons and industry. More recently this trend has linked up with the world-wide counterculture which is a response to the abuse of power and authority in our Western world.

Change over a period of seven years transformed a typical, hierarchical, rural mental hospital into a relatively open system. Portrayed is the unfolding of this change process within the hospital and our infiltration into the surrounding community of 100,000 people in the south of Scotland. Our enthusiasm for creating a holistic community mental health programme would spread, we hoped, by contagion and infect our surrounding environment with a positive attitude toward health. The description is as objective as possible, leaving the reader to assess for him/herself the extent and value of this change. Dingleton's story will be judged as a success by some and as an attack on the establishment and the traditional hierarchical hospital system by others.

BACKGROUND

Most of my professional life has been spent trying to understand how groups of people brought together for a specific purpose cannot only achieve their goal, but more importantly learn and grow along the way. Over the years it has become clear that, in fact, process actually takes precedence over goal achievement. For it is in the 'how' things are accomplished that the opportunity for learning and growth is present. I believe the kind of system described herein offers the optimal environment for growth.

My interest in groups began as a schoolboy in Edinburgh, where I realized the power of the peer group. I was elected captain of the school rugby team in my final year and, without consulting a soul, I arranged to play a team which on the surface was much too strong for us. I was severely criticized by our own school authorities for such bizarre independent action, but my team-mates relished the challenge to achieve the 'impossible'. We *had* to win and win we did with a comfortable margin!

Blessed with a gifted and liberal family and living in a country which for centuries had fought oppression from its much more

1

powerful neighbour (England), independence and freedom had a high priority in my value system. A group identity, whether home, school or country, far transcended the more universal values of money, power and material success. In this context medicine seemed to offer a humanely satisfying role in life. Having read widely in 'classical' literature with its preoccupation with understanding the nuances of character, I never doubted that the social and psychological had, for me, an appeal far stronger than physical disease. As far as I know, Edinburgh had the first professorship in family practice to be found any-where, and the whole cultural climate stressed service to society rather than monetary rewards - I received £50 for my first six months' post-graduate hospital work!

With this somewhat atypical approach to medicine - few people thought of mental health as a career in the 1920s - I suffered the horrors of a medical training and its relative insensitivity to the role of the patient. Worse still, the professors were on the whole coldly impersonal, dialogue and human relations were largely absent, and learning as a social process was entirely absent.

After graduation in 1931 I spent nine years following the pseudoscientific emphasis of academic psychiatry, first at the medical school in Edinburgh, and later at the Maudsley Hospital in London (probably the pre-eminent post-graduate psychiatric centre in Europe at that time). I published articles in the research fields of biochemistry, endocrinology, enzyme chemistry and various aspects of physiology.

The start of the Second World War proved to be my salvation. My interest in psychosomatic medicine resulted in my appointment to head a Maudsley Hospital team to study a condition known variously as Soldier's Heart, or Effort Syndrome, or in the USA as Neurocirculatory Asthenia.

This condition had resulted in large numbers of casualties in the First World War and had never been fully understood. The symptoms of left chest pain, breathlessness, postural giddiness, fainting and fatigue were doubtfully organic, and yet not clearly 'neurotic'. Intensive studies in exercise response in the bio-chemical and physiological fields, together with psychiatric evalu-ation, slowly uncovered the basic nature of the condition (Jones, 1948). Several years later when the USA entered the war, our results explaining this condition were largely confirmed by the Harvard Fatigue Laboratory.

What I want to stress is that our physiological and research findings in relation to Effort Syndrome were shared daily with a group of a hundred young soldiers who were able to realize that their supposed heart disease could be understood mechan-istically, for example, their left chest pain resulted from muscle tension in the intercostal muscles which disappeared if novocaine was injected into the intercostal muscles in the region of the heart, or by spinal root block. The rapid shallow breathing also characteristic of their condition was related to tension of the

diaphragmatic muscles easily demonstrated on the X-ray screen. These two factors contributed to the muscle pain inevitably resulting from continued spasm, and was recognized on the left side of the chest 'over the heart' as a consequence of their own subjective expectation. We were able to explain mechanistically their postural giddiness, fainting and their poor exercise tolerance.

This process of objectifying and externalizing their internal symptoms entirely changed their attitudes towards their symptoms – they no longer feared sudden death or permanent incapacity from heart disease. We helped them to share their knowledge with new referrals who almost invariably believed they were victims of heart disease. Many had seen cardiologists who, finding no organic disease, had told them they had nothing wrong with them, which made no sense in view of their symptomatology. For the first time as a doctor I experienced people living together in an environment which was not only conducive to treatment, but which could be studied and modified as well. In these five war years we moved from studying the physiology and biochemistry of fatigue to sharing research findings with the hundred patients in one large group (surely the first large group practice in the UK). This feedback of research material helped the men to 'objectify' their symptoms, which were no longer seen as some mysterious 'heart disease', but an eminently understandable physiological malfunction. Inevitably these large group meetings came to serve the purpose not only of discussing symptoms, but of information-sharing of social factors in the environment. My colleagues and I were being made aware of the social forces in the environment which could be utilized to effect attitude change. It amounted to patients treating patients, and anticipated by many years the current use of paramedics and ex-patients in treatment – especially with drug and alcohol abuse.

This period (1940-5), which might be described as a study of the physiology of change, was followed by an equally important experience in the sociology of change. In May 1945 I was asked to head a unit staffed from the Maudsley Hospital to rehabilitate the most disturbed of the 100,000 British prisoners of war returned from Europe and the Far East (Jones, 1952, pp. 15-24). This unit of 300 beds was in being for a year and gave us a wonderful opportunity to develop with six cottages, each housing fifty men. Daily cottage community meetings of all patients and staff helped them to work through their fears of impotence, inefficiency, and paranoid feelings in relation to their wives, former workmates, etc., resulting from up to five years' incarceration in prisoner-of-war camps. The patients were bussed daily to the 47 outside employments at which they chose to work, ranging from farms to factories. The timing was perfect as factory workers had made good money during the war while our patients had been POWs. This early example of a programme based on rehabilitation in a real-life setting effected significant changes in the men.

The war was now over and by great good fortune our experience with various aspects of change in social systems had a further stimulus when, as a result of our success in rehabilitating POWs, we were asked by the Ministries of Health and Labour to initiate a unit of one hundred beds for the rehabilitation of the 'hard core' unemployed in London. Britain had an outstanding record in the rehabilitation of the disabled unemployed, but it was well known that there was a significant group of unemployed people who defied ordinary diagnostic criteria, whether physical or mental, and yet seemed unable (or unwilling) to work. Here was another anomalous group in society which needed to be understood if they were to be 'treated'. And so almost totally unaware of the significance of our undertaking, we embarked on a study of character disorders in persons sometimes called sociopaths or psychopaths.

This was the beginning of what came to be known as the therapeutic community movement. Our clients were misfits in society and were avoided by almost everyone, including psychiatrists! They were as liable to end up in prison as in hospital, and even in the latter were often discriminated against. They covered the whole range of antisocial behaviour from passive dependent unemployed to crime and violence, through sexual aberrations to drugs and alcohol. Luckily the post-war climate in Britain was more favourable to social experiment than at any time before or since. Although the spirit of change and greater freedom was in the air, we inevitably met very strong resistance from our own profession and might never have survived but for the backing of leaders like Sir Aubrey Lewis, Professor of Psychiatry at the Postgraduate Medical School in London.

In the early years we felt very much alone, but with the growing influence of group treatment, family treatment and social psychiatry in the 1950s we slowly gained some credibility even with the medical profession. Later in the 1960s and 1970s the growth of systems theory as applied to social organizations in general resulted in most of our early findings being validated by developments in the behavioural sciences. Even in the more conservative area of physical medicine, the evolution of holistic medicine has been very much in line with our own philosophy.

The original therapeutic community which started in 1947 at Henderson Hospital near London is still in existence. I was director from 1947 until 1959, then moved to the United States, first as visiting professor at Stanford University for a year, and then as Director of Education and Research at Oregon State Hospital in Salem, Oregon, from 1960 to 1962. There we developed a therapeutic community in a large state hospital and began to explore the possibilities of community mental health services expanding into the surrounding community.

The circumstances leading to my departure typified the risks inherent in the role of a change agent. Although the project in Oregon was an important pioneering development in social psychiatry, antedating the Community Mental Health Act of the

Kennedy Administration (1963), it aroused strong resistance in this conservative state. It was made expedient for me to leave! There was no hint of personal animosity, but we became the target of political pressure. These events circulated on the grapevine and I was offered better-paying posts in more liberal states, but preferred to return to Scotland. It is significant that the interest generated by therapeutic community ideas in the USA influenced the treatment philosophy of Fort Logan Mental Health Center. This was a new state hospital started in 1961 and designed to meet the needs of approximately a million people living in Denver, Colorado. We were visited in Oregon by Dr Al Kraft and colleagues who were planning the new state hospital in Colorado. It became what was probably the outstanding example of an open system in the USA and I was to spend five years there at a later date.

MY ARRIVAL AT DINGLETON HOSPITAL

Professor Morris Carstairs, then head of the Department of Psychiatry at Edinburgh University, encouraged me to return from Oregon to my native land and this I was glad to do. He pointed out the advantages of a rural hospital which served a relatively small population with very little mobility. I was familiar with Dingleton from the past and liked what Dr George Bell, my predecessor, had accomplished in creating the first totally open mental hospital in the English-speaking world. This he achieved in 1949, before the advent of tranquillizers.

Thus, in 1962 I returned to Scotland as the Superintendent of Dingleton Hospital in Melrose, 35 miles south of Edinburgh. Melrose is a small town of 2,000 inhabitants. The River Tweed flows through this beautiful countryside and gave its name to the cloth manufactured in the mills in the small towns of this area.

The most difficult part of the process of change (Jones, 1968a, pp. 19-22) was my initial impact with an established traditional psychiatric hospital. Like a stepfather joining his new family, I had to become known as a person and then incorporated within the family structure before one could even think about harmonious relationships. I arrived at Dingleton on 10 December 1962, with a clear idea of what I wanted to do. I had spent the major part of my professional career working on the concept of a therapeutic community. This had come to mean that the people involved have an opportunity to interact, listen, learn, plan, evolve and grow in a way that reflects their own individual and collective capability and potential. The dynamic comes in part from the social organization of such a unit, plus the motivation of the people involved. I wanted to test out these principles in a suitable setting and Dingleton seemed to offer an ideal opportunity. (Another part of my reason for choosing to go to Dingleton was that my critics always said that the therapeutic community was fine for psychopaths, but would not be appropriate for other

kinds of patients.) I had grown up in Edinburgh and knew the
Border country; a population of 100,000 was distributed among
the counties of Berwickshire, Selkirkshire and Roxburghshire,
and the mental health needs of these people were served by
Dingleton Hospital.

Although I had a theoretical framework and a long-term goal,
I knew that to impose preconceived ideas on a hospital population
without their involvement was to antagonize and insult the people
concerned. I knew of the need to establish two-way communication
and decision-making machinery at all levels. Experience had
taught me that if this could be achieved, then a process of
evolution was started; but where it would lead could not be pre-
dicted with any certainty. Anyone interested in the theoretical
basis on which we operated is referred to separate accounts
(Jones, 1952; 1962; 1968a; 1968b; 1976a).

PRINCIPAL CHARACTERS

The leaders at Dingleton when I arrived were the Deputy
Physician Superintendent, Dr Ken Morrice; the Matron, Miss
Mullen; and the Hospital Secretary/Treasurer, Jimmy Millar.
These people all gave permission for their real names to be used,
having read the manuscript. In some instances reference is made
to individuals not on the staff at Dingleton and here pseudonyms
are used. Ken was a colourful Celt from Aberdeen, a strange
mixture of charm, intelligence and inscrutability. A well-trained
psychiatrist, he had a very clear idea about the function and
importance of a consultant and had, I think, some difficulty in
relinquishing his professional role to become submerged in a
peer group. He had visited Henderson Hospital in London, where
he was greatly impressed by the possibilities of this democratic
approach and was already beginning to initiate such developments
at Dingleton. He had been on the staff for five years before my
arrival, and he had applied unsuccessfully for the post of Superintendent, which I had òbtained. He could not have been more
generous about this potentially difficult situation and was out-
spokenly in favour of the therapeutic community approach. In
addition, as a person of immense integrity, time and again he
questioned my interpretation of the process of change. I undoubtedly owe him a great deal for his circumspection, his canny
Aberdonian fear of exploitation, and his readiness to become
involved and openly challenge my position and ideas.

He inevitably became the leader of the opposition; we had many
painful interludes until other leaders began to emerge, but with
multiple leadership in a multidisciplinary setting our discord
began to look much more like a learning process than interpersonal rivalry. His value as an exponent of therapeutic community
principles and practice was amply demonstrated when he spent
a sabbatical year (1966) at Fort Logan Mental Health Center in
Denver, Colorado. There he was highly regarded and made a

valuable contribution during his stay. Ken is something of a mystic and writes and publishes extremely good poetry. Although I like and respect him, I cannot honestly say that I fully understand him, but that is part of his charm.

Miss Mullen, the Matron, is another extraordinary and admirable person. When I first met her she seemed to epitomize the power of the nursing profession: a massive presence, the embodiment of authority, one's first reaction was one of awe. The minute she began to interact this impression was modified, because she became a feeling, sensitive and intelligent colleague. Nevertheless, I never quite got over my feeling of awe, and unfortunately, she kept this alive by periodic explosions of anger, which one simply had to accept as part of her Irish personality. At her best, she was a delightful, entertaining and humorous person. At her worst, she was frankly intimidating. She had immense integrity and was able to be remarkably honest with herself. She deplored the fact that at times she was her own worst enemy, saying in anger things which she regretted in retrospect. We worked together with periodic episodes of harmony and discord, but I never lost my respect for her and her unrelenting protection of 'her own' nursing department at Dingleton. Having reached the top of her profession, my arrival suddenly confronted her with a completely new set of expectations which undermined many of her professional values established over a lifetime. That she went along with so many changes and actively contributed to the whole process of change is indeed a remarkable tribute to her as a human being. Like a person who is courageous despite uncertainty and fear, she associated herself with a development which caused her probably more anguish than any other single person on the Dingleton staff. We even published a paper together (Jones and Mullen, 1963).

Jimmy Millar, the Hospital Secretary and Treasurer, was a delight to me from the start. He shared my liking for the drama of a situation and seemed intuitively to respond to the possibility of a hospital community which reflected the ideas and personalities of the people in it. He was born and bred within a few miles of Dingleton and took pride in the fact that he belonged to the same world from which the majority of patients came. Time and time again he acted as my interpreter so that I could better understand the local culture. In fact, I came to the point where I would not put a step outside Dingleton in my professional role without first consulting him. He was, I suppose, if such a thing exists, the typical Borderer, but quite atypical was his willingness to change in the light of increased understanding and learning. This almost 'psychopathic' detachment from the mores of his culture which gave him his unique flexibility was all the more remarkable because of his civil service upbringing. To have such a colleague and friend for my own 'intelligent delinquency' was, I think, the greatest single factor in allowing us to change to the extent that we did.

I must mention one other highly significant person during the

first half of my stay at Dingleton. One could say that Dingleton had strong representation from the 'good old days' as long as Dr Winifred Small reigned with us. She, like Matron, was called on to make an almost superhuman change if she was to meet the new expectations. No one knew Dingleton, its patients and nurses, as well or as intimately as Dr Small. Legend and, I think, fact combined to picture her running Dingleton during the Second World War almost singlehandedly. Not surprisingly, without any formal psychiatric training and with a general practice background, she had come to develop her own rule-of-thumb methods for running an understaffed mental hospital. Her dedication was heroic, but also a damned nuisance because one felt guilty in asking her to be less ubiquitous. Both in Dingleton and in the outside community, people had learned to turn to her in any psychiatric emergency. She had learned how to cope in a highly individualistic and effective way. She relieved the urgent anxiety of a family doctor seeking immediate admission for one of his patients, day or night. She took over the role of arbiter of right and wrong and decided everything for everyone. You either operated with her or were alienated. Matron and other authority figures who refused to conform to Dr Small's ideas had to be excluded from her system, so that at least two systems operated in Dingleton: the system that had evolved over years and had great effectiveness when controlled completely by Dr Small; and a much less organized and frustrated opposition led by Matron. Realizing Dr Small's immense influence, power and value, we tried to integrate her, at least loosely, within a therapeutic community system. Not surprisingly Dr Small never conceded more than a token acknowledgment of therapeutic community principles. When she finally retired in September 1966 I had lost none of my respect and affection for this irascible woman, but like most of the staff felt a deep sense of relief! In a funny way, both she and Matron, although barely on speaking terms, protected the interests of the old guard and constantly reminded those of us who were interested in the development of a therapeutic community that there were other models - in particular, the traditional hierarchical hospital.

I have dwelt on these four people at some length because this is essentially an account of people and how they interact in a setting which calls for the pooling of interest and effort. The first half of my stay reflected the impact of therapeutic community principles on 'ordinary' professional people. The hierarchical structure of the hospital was threatened and, very understandably, leaders were found to protect the status quo. Dr Small and many people who had worked and lived in Dingleton for years before I came represented this stand. Dr Ken Morrice wanted the hospital to change, but circumstances found him playing the role of leader of the opposition, and no democratic evolution is possible without a competent and articulate opposition party. Ken, in my opinion, made a significant contribution to Dingleton's growth. The same can be said about Matron, although for her

change presented personality difficulties which required an almost heroic effort to overcome. Jimmy Millar had a potential which came to light as the new social organization evolved.

SYSTEMS THEORY AND THERAPEUTIC COMMUNITIES

The concept of a therapeutic community means different things to different people. It can be seen as being a part of systems theory in general. The term 'social system' refers to a consistent network of interacting relationships between persons, with the persons considered as units of the system above and beyond their individual characteristics. One looks at a group of people not in terms of their individual personalities, but as people having certain positions and tasks within the network. One looks at the relationships *between* these units, rather than at each unit as an independent entity (Murrell, 1973, p. 9). Alternatively, a system is viewed as an organized whole unit which includes the inter- actions of its interdependent component parts, and its relation- ship to the environment (Buckley, 1967).

We are concerned here primarily with systems that are 'open' and that interact readily with their environment, both physical and social, and are therefore open to new learning and growth. Growth can be thought of as the process by which things become connected with each other and operate at higher levels of organ- ization and complexity. We return to this topic in the Epilogue.

I am now of the opinion that the term 'therapeutic community' has served a useful purpose in drawing attention to the need for democratization in hospital settings. It is, however, better thought of in the wider context of open systems. This avoids much of the controversy, which to me appears rather unprofit- able, as to what is the real meaning of a therapeutic community. There is no such thing as 'the' therapeutic community (or a totally 'open' system), but merely attempts in varying ways under different circumstances with different people and differing ideol- ogies to introduce open system theories to the practice in mental hospitals or any other facilities.

Another controversial issue surrounds the term 'therapeutic'. Treatment brings to mind the doctor-patient relationship and the various theories surrounding psychoanalytic and other methods of treatment. With the proliferation of endless cults, all of which claim to be therapeutic, it seems time that we began to look at all these varying phenomena in terms of learning as a social process.

In my most recent book (1976a, pp. 43-53) I have referred to social learning as two-way communication in a group of individuals motivated by some inner need or stress leading to overt or covert expression of feeling and involving cognitive processes and change. The term implies a change in the individual's attitude and/or beliefs as a result of the experience. These changes are incorporated and modify his personality and self-image.

The concept of social learning is referred to repeatedly in the

following chapters. Put alongside accepted treatment modalities, such as the various types of psychotherapy, behaviour modification, transactional analysis, etc., it has, I think, achieved the right to be called a methodology. But like all other methodologies, it cannot stand alone but must borrow from whatever techniques appear to be relevant in any particular situation. Equally, other treatment techniques must utilize social learning if they are to be optimally (holistically) effective. In Chapter 8 I attempt a synthesis of the process of change over my seven years at Dingleton with special reference to social learning.

Starting with a fairly typical hierarchical hospital system we achieved a relatively open system which harmonized with many other aspects of the outside community. This included our impact on local government, schools and family doctors in our catchment area. I am convinced that this study of a microcosm of society is a valid model for social systems in general.

The content is largely descriptive, based on a weekly diary which I kept over the seven years. The diary was built on the minutes of the Senior Staff Committee recorded faithfully by my secretary, Cathy. These minutes were fed back the following day to the SSC and therefore reflect the consensus of the whole group. Each of seven chapters chronologically covers one of the seven years and is summarized with particular reference to the learning and change process.

Chapter 1

The first year, 1963:
initiating a therapeutic community
in a closed system

INTRODUCTION

When I came to take up my post at Dingleton Hospital in December
1962, I found the traditional hierarchical structure of a 400-bed
British mental hospital. My predecessor, Dr George Bell, and
the Matron (Director of Nursing), Miss Mullen, both perceived
their roles in terms of status and authority. They showed little
or no tendency to bring about decision-making by consensus,
and unilateral decisions were a commonplace. The Deputy
Physician Superintendent, Dr Ken Morrice, who remained in
post, had been at Dingleton for five years before my arrival.
Although he had attempted to liberalize the social organization
by introducing more democratic procedures, his efforts had met
with little success. The role relationships between this doctor,
my predecessor and the Matron were far from satisfactory, and
communication had largely broken down. The Hospital Secretary,
Jimmy Millar, had acted as a go-between for my predecessor
and the Board of Management, and tended to identify with the
Physician Superintendent rather than the other hospital personnel.

My first concern was to establish two-way communication and
decision-making machinery at all levels of the hospital organization. My goal (desired future state of affairs) was, as already
stated, to bring about a social environment for creative fulfilment by fostering learning as a social process. From my previous
experience in developing five therapeutic communities in hospitals
since 1940, I had certain expectations about the validity of open
system principles and practice in effecting change in the desired
direction. In retrospect, I can see the evolution of change in a
series of stages. For those readers interested in theory I have
made references throughout the book to my previous publications.

THE HOSPITAL CULTURE IN DECEMBER 1962

My first concern was to become conversant with the existing
social structure, to study the roles, role relationships and the
overall culture of the people working and being treated in Dingleton Hospital. From the beginning I decided to keep a weekly
account called 'Impressions of Dingleton Hospital' and this was
maintained. This record of approximately 1500 words each week
gave me descriptive historical data for use in an attempt to

understand something of the process of change over the years.
The validity of this subjective account is open to question, but
this limitation is partly offset by the minutes of the Senior Staff
Committee. This record, compiled by Cathy Wilson, a most competent secretary, was corrected as the minutes of the previous
meeting were read out for approval or disapproval, and thus
reflects the opinion of the senior staff as accurately as possible.
In my first report written the week after my arrival I note:

> My predecessor does not seem to have had anything in the way
> of regular staff meetings, and in fact the conference room
> next door to my office seems to be almost completely unused.
> The single psychiatric social worker, aged 64, told me that
> she was seldom made use of by the doctors and her office was
> in a very remote part of the hospital. Two of the doctors, Ken
> Morrice and Raymond Ratcliffe, had started the first bi-weekly
> ward meetings with their patients, but these were not followed
> by a review session, and staff training seemed to be largely
> neglected. It seemed fairly clear that the nurses had only a
> limited idea of feedback and none regarding the importance of
> here-and-now situations for training. The hospital had no
> psychologist, and as yet no out-patient clinics had been
> developed in the community of 100,000 people which Dingleton
> served. A remarkable feature of the hospital was that since
> 1949, before the introduction of tranquillizing drugs, my pre-
> decessor, Dr George Bell, had maintained an entirely open
> hospital, the first of its kind in the present century in Britain
> or the USA.

STAGE 1   INTRODUCTION OF TWO-WAY COMMUNICATION
AND DECISION-MAKING MACHINERY

Weeks one to three
Three weeks after my arrival I noted many areas of discontent
and acrimony between the heads of the nursing staff and the
medical staff. We had initiated a bi-weekly Senior Staff Meeting
with the Hospital Secretary, the four senior nurses, the five
doctors (including myself), the psychiatric social worker, my
secretary and other senior staff personnel. I went on to note:

> The Matron has come to one ward meeting so far and seems to
> be quite interested. She has also agreed to the establishment
> of a monthly over-all staff meeting where any of her nursing
> personnel, and in fact any staff who have contact with patients,
> are to be invited. We have also initiated a monthly Journal Club
> meeting for all staff. The female admission ward is having a
> daily ward meeting with all five doctors attending. The com-
> munication network is being improved and the system of uni-
> lateral decision-making is being modified. There seems, at this
> stage, to be no resistance to the ideas of democratic decision-

making in preference to the unilateral decision-making process.
The Hospital Secretary, Jimmy Millar, is coming to the Senior
Staff Meeting twice a week and seems prepared to participate
in any of the ongoing programmes.

I noted the tensions in the top administration and the relative
absence of open communication or an integrated programme. The
result was a kind of cell-like quality in the hospital with little
evidence of links between the various activities and departments.
From what has been said it is apparent that within three weeks
of my arrival at Dingleton we had already begun to change the
social organization of the hospital, particularly in relation to
information-sharing, two-way communication and decision-making.
Some people might see this as imprudent, but in retrospect I
feel that the rapid introduction of new ideas fitted in with the
expectations of my role by the more articulate leaders in the
hospital. Everyone seemed ready for change but no one knew
quite how to initiate this. The fact that there were only 400 beds
in the hospital with a comparatively small staff of five doctors,
84 nurses, one psychiatric social worker, etc., made the establish
ment of better communications relatively easy.

Weeks four to eight
At the end of four weeks the first meeting of the Work Therapy
Subcommittee had been held. This subcommittee included the
Hospital Secretary, the social worker, two doctors, three senior
nurses, the occupational therapist, the recreational therapist
and the supervisors in the areas of the laundry, gardens,
kitchen and dining-room, all of whom had patients working with
them. I recorded:

> It looks as though this committee will be in session for many
> months. Its function is to make recommendations to the Senior
> Staff Committee and to bring about an integration of all the
> activity programmes. The questions of graded stages of re-
> habilitation, the nature of the activity programme, pay, the na-
> ture of patient referral, the extent of doctor involvement and
> the feedback to the treatment team are all under consideration.

At the end of four weeks the first meeting of the Hospital Discussion Group had been held:

> This is to take place on the first Monday of the month at 7.45 p.m.
> and is voluntary. For the first meeting approximately sixty
> people turned up, mainly nurses, but also representatives of
> the tradesmen and the various patient activity groups. All the
> doctors and senior nurses were present. It seems to me that it
> was a very productive meeting. There was, perhaps luckily,
> the usual discontented aggressive nurse. Reg Elliott
> provides an example of a risk-taker throughout this book
> (see Chapter 8, p. 147), who talked about the frustration

and futility of nursing as it was practised at this hospital. He said that he had heard about teamwork before and that it was just a name. He gave quite good illustrations of the lack of importance accorded to the nursing role in the hospital, and was backed by several other nurses. The main complaint was that they were not allowed to share an interest in the clinical work and were not even given access to the case notes. This led to a spirited discussion about the nurses' involvement in teamwork and I pointed out that the admission ward had already established an admission procedure where two of the nurses, the social worker, the new patient, a relative and myself all met together. We then discussed the problem that the patient presented and what the treatment goal ought to be.

At the end of the first month my role as Superintendent was coming in for some discussion (Jones, 1968a, pp. 23-9). I felt that one of the best ways to encourage the development of a democratic structure was to establish a role model of this type myself. I agreed to have new patients referred to me by my medical colleagues; in this way I ensured that I would have a certain number of patients distributed throughout the hospital, and so would be in a position to share the difficulties of patient management with all the personnel and patients in these areas. Thus far my role relationship with all the senior staff had been excellent. I was well aware of the fact that this was partly due to my newness and that the 'honeymoon' could not last for ever. In particular, the two most senior nurses, Matron and her deputy, had felt isolated and rejected by the majority of the hospital at the time of my arrival. I note:

I think they are grateful to have a sympathetic listener which at the moment I find a reasonable and compatible thing to do. They have agreed, without demur, to the establishment of a nursing committee, although they must realize that this portends a big change in the authority structure. They have both now become members of treatment groups.

My diary continues:

The first meeting of the Journal Club was held last Thursday evening. Between fifty and sixty staff turned up which must have represented a very large percentage of all staff who were available to attend. The three senior doctors and their wives and the nursing personnel were also present, as were the two junior doctors. At my suggestion we discussed Denis Martin's very interesting account of the development of the therapeutic community at Claybury Hospital near London entitled 'Adventure in Psychiatry' [Martin, 1962]. This, I think, was a happy choice because Martin's book is very simply written and describes the early stages of his experimental ward in developing a community approach. The discussion was fairly brief, but

one of the staff nurses said that she herself had already bought the book. Later I learned that another of the nurses had done so and they both enjoyed reading it.

Despite this promising start we soon learned that reading was to play no significant part in our growth. Learning by direct involvement together with frequent group discussions quickly replaced reading as an educational approach.

The numerous meetings we have now established in the hospital are tending to bud off, so that subcommittees are developing and group meetings are spreading to other wards. Moreover, the communication network seems to be linking up very satisfactorily with the Hospital Board of Management. They now know that recommendations made to them have been discussed already in the Senior Staff Committee, if not in other subcommittees before that. They are not only getting my point of view but that of the senior staff generally. In addition, it has now been agreed that the doctors can have representation in the Board of Management through a separate medical subcommittee if they so desire it. They also have the right to appear personally before the board at any time, so they do not have only the Physician Superintendent speaking for them. The Board of Management has agreed to a one-way screen for teaching purposes, to the employment of a second psychiatric social worker, and indeed have so far supported every proposition put up by the staff.

The Work Therapy Subcommittee is progressing very well indeed. It looks as though we will not need to go outside the hospital to look for work. This may be one advantage of a small rural hospital, in that we seem to have adequate work to be done without seeking subcontracted work from outside. We have yet to mend various items from the laundry which need repair. We do all the laundry work for other hospitals in the Borders and process well over a million articles a year so that there is a big job waiting to be done here. As yet nothing has been done to employ patients on a large scale in the laundry. This would require supervision from the nurses in order to make it both therapeutic and functional. The nursing staff accept the concept that a work role alongside patients is therapeutically desirable.

Another new topic is the absence of a patients' canteen. This has been in the background for years, but it has now been agreed by the Hospital Board of Management that we can go ahead and organize one. We made a plea that we should allow this to be run by the patients as far as possible, and that we should only call for help from the Red Cross or other voluntary groups if it was absolutely necessary. We felt this would give the patients a much greater feeling of identity with the project, and supply responsible roles for them to play while still in hospital.

Three months later the canteen was in fact opened and run largely by the patients.

By the end of the two months, the Senior Staff Committee had established itself as an important democratic administrative decision-making body integrating well with the Board of Management, and with Jimmy Millar, the Hospital Secretary, as a valuable liaison to both bodies and attending all their meetings.

In the first two months, I had made contact with four of the family doctors, and got the impression that Dingleton was seen as a valuable resource by these doctors. We had begun to have patients' wives attending ward groups on the male admission ward. I had made contact with the officials of the local Red Cross with a view to greater involvement with the community, and requesting volunteers from the outside to help in the geriatric wards, etc. The volunteer programme did not flourish until five years later, when we recruited a paid co-ordinator.

The first two months might be called the 'honeymoon phase'. I felt welcome, and because of a prior interest in groups and in the concept of a therapeutic community by some of the senior staff, there was an apparent readiness for change. It seemed that the senior staff's expectations of my role and my own idea regarding my function were complementary. There were, however, many factors which I could only be aware of marginally, or which escaped me altogether. At the highest level of the hospital organization the desire for change in the direction of a more democratic egalitarian structure was already present and presented me with a ready-made catalytic function. How people would actually like the changes when effected was not measurable as the time period was too short. Moreover, interpersonal problems were bound to develop in any group of people working together toward a common goal. Again, it took time for these problems to become overt. The social organization, with emphasis on two-way communication and the establishment of a decision-making machinery at all levels, seemed to me to have gone surprisingly well during these first two months. However, I was aware of the vast area, particularly in relation to the patient population and the nurses generally, with whom I had not yet had time to make any real contact. It was in the long-stay where most of the patients and staff were to be found, that institutionalized patterns were most apparent. Some of the nurses had been in charge of their wards for periods of up to twenty years, and it was too much to expect that the patterns of a lifetime would respond readily to change.

The senior staff, who knew something about the concept of a therapeutic community (and on the whole were eager to try it out), were much better prepared for my arrival than were the junior staff, who knew little or nothing of these ideas. Moreover, the senior staff were, of course, anxious to make a good im-

pression on me and to gain my approval. At this period, three months after my arrival, resistance from the nursing staff began to be spearheaded by a male nurse, Reg, who was both articulate and intelligent:

> On Wednesday we had our first meeting, from 3.00 to 4.00 p.m., with the nurses. This was intended in time to involve every nurse in the hospital for one hour so that they could have an opportunity of discussing the way in which the goals of a therapeutic community affected them. At this meeting, the now familiar male nurses' fear that they were going to be displaced by other categories of staff was voiced. In this context the arrival of Jim, in a new role to integrate the activity groups, was discussed. The function of the various hospital committees were outlined. Reg Elliott intervened to say that the Nursing Subcommittee had not been democratically elected, but had been chosen by the administration. I felt bound to say that he was right, but added that if they could not have confidence in the ten senior administrators and their judgement in selecting people to represent them, then it raised the whole question of how far they really could believe in the hospital at all. There had been some talk of an election and I wondered if we were yet ready for such a procedure until the whole hospital became more aware of the meaning of the democratic process. [In retrospect this sounds distinctly manipulative!] Reg then raised the question of the confidentiality of these meetings and cited an instance where one of the night staff had heard that he had been discussed and that he was going to be transferred to another ward. I said that I thought we were talking about Nurse Jenkins and we then described exactly what happened – a transfer due to staff shortage. Unfortunately, Matron got somewhat angry with Reg, and I felt it was necessary to point out that he really did take a delight in making authority figures feel uncomfortable. He might be seen as telling us more about himself than about the actual event. People laughed at this and it become apparent that it was better at times to see the nursing meetings as serving a learning as well as an information-sharing function.

n retrospect this seems a poor use of Reg's risk-taking role Jones, 1976a, pp. 38-43). It would seem that because of my nsecurity I felt the need to support the authority structure.

STAGE 2   THE SECOND THREE MONTHS

Widening parameters – extramural developments
On 24 April 1963, I met the three Medical Officers of Health who represented the public health interests of the counties of Ber-wickshire, Roxburghshire, Selkirkshire and Peeblesshire:

The Medical Health Officers had lunch with us and stayed
until about 2.30. My aim was to try to see if the three health
officers would collaborate and share a psychiatrist and social
worker among them, whose salaries would be paid by the local
authority. It soon became clear that Dr Sawyer in particular
felt this was quite unworkable because the local authority
could pay nothing comparable to the salary the National Health
Service would pay a consultant psychiatrist, and he felt that
anyone less than a consultant would have little or no acceptance with the local general practitioners. In any case, he felt
that a consultant employed at Dingleton would have much more
status than a consultant employed at the local authority. I
stressed the fact that the most important role that a consultant
could play would be to educate existing personnel in the local
authority. This task would apply not only to the psychiatrist
but to the social worker. It was agreed that some local authorities in Britain had employed their own psychiatrists but
these were the exception. The Medical Officers of Health would
be glad if they could get new welfare officers who were well
trained and send them to Dingleton for a month or two before
starting work. They also would be glad to avail themselves of
any programme for their district nurses and could spare them
for a week at a time to attend a course at Dingleton. The
officers said that they felt competent enough to decide about
the minor degrees of mental deficiency, but completely incom-
petent in dealing with psychiatric cases. They felt that if a
psychiatrist and social worker were available for consultation
from Dingleton, they would not need more than a monthly
clinic in towns like Duns, Peebles, or even Hawick. They all
seemed to favour the idea of multidisciplinary training seminar
possibly in the form of a case conference at such a clinic.

The meeting was extremely interesting and taught me a lot,
but at the same time it was rather depressing. It became perfectly clear that the local authority were not likely to recogniz
officially the unique opportunity that the Borders offered for
a first-class mental health service, and that initiative and
extra staffing would in all probability have to come from us
in the first instance. Local authorities were quite likely to act
at a later date provided they had some evidence that additiona
personnel would be a sound investment. Dr Inglis, one of the
Medical Officers of Health, suggested that if we could provide
50 per cent of the money to pay a consultant psychiatrist, the
local authority might then be induced to pay the other 50 per
cent.

One important point discussed was the possibility of inform-
ing the local authority in every case of a patient discharged
from hospital. It might be adequate if we simply sent a copy
of the letter sent to the general practitioner to the local
authority. The Medical Officers of Health felt that this would
be most useful, but would prefer if we would first ask the
patients if they would agree to a home visit when necessary

by one of the local authority personnel. They felt that it was more appropriate that we should ask permission before the patient's discharge rather than make the overtures themselves. In fact, if permission was granted, this could be incorporated in the letter to the general practitioner so that everyone would be kept informed about what was happening.

Two months later in my 'Impressions' of 7 June 1963, I wrote:

The developments with the community have gone extremely well. We had a meeting with the three Medical Officers of Health yesterday and we seemed to have a complete agreement about the need to develop a positive programme for the Borders. It seems highly probable that the counties of Roxburghshire, Selkirkshire and Berwickshire will, among them, supply one psychiatric social worker. There was full agreement that the social worker should be located near Dingleton, and if possible even have a house supplied by us. This is geographically and operationally expedient for both parties.

Hospital - intramural developments
The idea of a similar cafeteria menu for staff and patients came up for discussion. At the fourth monthly meeting open to all hospital staff on Monday evening, 1 April 1963, I recorded:

There was a large turn-out of approximately fifty hospital personnel representing all the different activities within the hospital. Most of the time was spent discussing the hospital plans to change both the diet and the physical setting for eating. We hope to have the same food for both the patients and the staff, offering a choice of meals as suggested by a Scottish Health Service Report. In addition, we would like to have all the patients' meals served between twelve noon and one o'clock and then have the nurses' meal times co-ordinated to fit with this pattern. There was a good deal of feeling expressed about eating with the patients. The nursing staff said that they were with them all day and needed a break. It was discussed and nearly conceded that we would not have any mixing of the staff and patients, but that circumstances might require that some of them ate at the same time. Tom, a ward orderly, pointed out that it would be very hard on the kitchen staff to carry out such a programme unless they had a great deal more help from patients. To have a choice of dishes for the patients meant an enormous amount of extra work. I suggested that some of this shortage of staff could be met by closing the dining-room upstairs in the doctors' quarters as well as the separate staff dining-room.

Matron and her deputy dined in state like royalty in their own quarters, and the staff dining-room had the exclusiveness of a London club. This reminds me of my amazement on my first day

in office when my secretary, Cathy, appeared with an impressive
tea tray for my exclusive enjoyment - all apparently a part of the
existing feudal culture. Cathy's relief at my surprise was delight
ful and we both giggled about the situation.

On 1 April the patients' canteen was opened and run as a
patient activity. About the same time we initiated a news-sheet
which was handed out weekly to all staff when they were paid
and copies were sent to all the wards so that the patients were
kept informed about hospital activities, visitors, changes in
policy and so on. In my 'Impressions of Dingleton Hospital' at
the end of eighteen weeks, 13 April 1963, I noted:

> The most important thing that has happened this week has
> been the preoccupation with limit setting for patient behaviour
> At their meeting the nurses seem to think that ten o'clock is
> the time when patients are supposed to have returned to their
> wards, but many people are ignorant of this fact. Matron said
> firmly that it is a rule. The question of lateness came to a hea(
> because of the acting-out behaviour, particularly in the female
> ward. Two female patients had been out one evening until
> 11.30 p.m. and caused considerable anxiety about possible
> activity. The younger people in the female admission ward
> talked about the dullness of the ward on weekends and wanted
> to have permission to attend a dance on the day of the Melrose
> Rugby Seven-a-Side Sports, Saturday, 13 April. We heard
> reports from the male admission ward that patients were gettin
> the idea that they could do what they liked sexually and that
> Dr Jones was sanctioning all kinds of freedom.

By the beginning of May 1963 there seemed to be growing evidence of a more tolerant attitude between staff and patients.
Feelings of security by patients resulting in freer communication
and a greater willingness to express feelings directly to authorit
figures produced problems. The doctors and senior nursing staf
were beginning to feel more threatened by the growing tendency
of patients and junior staff to question what we were doing and
why. My relationship with Matron epitomized this growing problem. We began to examine her position in relation to the catering
establishment and various other aspects of her role which had
developed over the years in an authoritarian system. We understandably made her feel threatened. She felt that we expected
her to change, and indeed this was perfectly true. Our attitude
and that of the nursing profession generally, was that senior
nurses should concern themselves with nursing, leaving housekeeping and other activities to other departments. However,
even at times of greatest stress in terms of our relationship, I
felt that we were both putting the hospital interests first, althou(
seeing many situations from completely different points of view.
Our capacity to interact never completely broke down. As the
senior staff grew in understanding and skill, so our capacity to
listen and learn from different points of view became more eviden

Inevitably, my own role had come in for a great deal of discussion, misunderstanding and rumour (Jones, 1968a, pp. 57-60). By the middle of May I noted:

Rumour has started to play its part in relation to my role. The laundry supervisor has talked about her somewhat flirtatious interludes with me in a way which has started a great deal of talk. I have tried to see her so that we could bring it out in the open for discussion; but she is so busy that she will not stop her work in the laundry, and blocks any approach to a discussion. I think she has many problems and feels overworked and understaffed, despite the high degree of automation which has been achieved in the laundry. She is a valuable supervisor and we feel that everything should be done to help her, but she makes this difficult. The most interesting part of the rumour is that I am said to be in a rivalry situation with one of the male student nurses. Actually the lady in question is extremely attractive and has a very important place in the social organization of Dingleton. She manages to attract most of the men, and I think I have been rather stupid in allowing any kind of situation to develop.

This brings us to the end of the first six months of my stay at Dingleton. It is extremely difficult to assess the position regarding the forces of reaction. They are undoubtedly strong but how strong I do not know. They are continually activated by Dr Small who tends to reinforce the inevitable anxiety which accompanies change. A good example of this was the meeting the senior nurses and doctors hold regularly with the night staff once a month. This meeting was attended by the night staff and by Dr Small and Dr Ratcliffe. Dr Small, addressing the night staff, said: 'We don't know where we are, do we? If a patient is out late and we reprimand her, all we are told is that Dr Jones says that she can do what she likes. Isn't this true?' Dr Small said, turning to the nurses. Dr Small makes no secret of the fact that this is how she reinforces the nurses' anxieties, by implying that I will get very angry if my instructions are not carried out. Needless to say, my instructions have never encouraged any laxity of self-control; this confusion between permissiveness and lack of discipline has been tightened up and we have had a formal ten o'clock ward rule now for some time.

The issue of permissiveness and licence created problems for many months and will be referred to again, as this was part of an evolutionary process. This demonstrates the differences between a hierarchical or closed system and a more democratic or open system. In the former rules are made and issued by the administration in response to problems which in no way represent the outcome of discussion and shared decision-making. In the latter everyone is involved in the decision-making process so that the rules become *their* rules with which they are

identified and feel responsible.

So far our problems have been confined to the hospital personnel, but some of the staff are beginning to convey rumours
outside. The one that has come up recently is the danger of
pregnancy and the myth that I am in favour of the abolition of
discipline. Jimmy Millar, the Hospital Secretary, assures me
that his contacts with the local police and other local figures
indicates no negative image developing in the general public.
Having now withdrawn from both admission wards and
operating entirely in the long-stay wards, I now attend five
ward meetings in different wards per week. This, plus the
weekly meeting with the charge nurses, the monthly meeting
with the total hospital staff, the Journal Club, the meeting
with the night nurses, and the standing committees total a
fair degree of contact with the hospital personnel.

STAGE 3 MONTHS SIX TO TWELVE

Staff - the changing culture
By the beginning of July 1963 we were having regular weekly
seminars for separate groups of charge nurses, staff nurses
and student nurses. These discussions were about any anxieties
to do with their work at Dingleton. These seminars were for me
an important communication link with the rest of the hospital in
relation to both patients and staff. The night nurses were beginning to feel left out of things and this was expressed at one of
their monthly meetings held in July:

The meeting this week with the night nurses was much more
positive than any of the monthly meetings held so far. The
nurses showed an interest in the hospital activities and felt
they were being left out of interesting developments. There
was some talk about an eight-hour shift of a rotating kind so
that they could get back into the swim of things. [At this time
the night nurses did permanent night duty on twelve-hour
shifts.] They also expressed some concern about the changing
hospital policy as it affected the mixing of the sexes and permissiveness generally. We discussed the importance of feedback
channels so that we could be kept informed about behaviour at
night and vice versa. The real control of deviant behaviour
came from the patients themselves. Public opinion among the
patients was probably the strongest and most effective
deterrent we could use. There was also some mention of the
way in which some of the staff were behaving, particularly a
student nurse and a married male nurse. The important thing
seemed to be that the night nurses want to be in a situation to
learn and to catch up with the current treatment developments

Informal learning was occurring with increasing frequency

whenever an opportunity, such as a crisis, presented itself. Socio-drama was also being used as a training device. In the middle of July at one of their meetings, the student nurses said that, like some of the senior nurses, they would like to be in- volved in home visits to ex-patients. By setting up a role-playing situation in an imaginary home we were able to demonstrate the difficulties which might be encountered when the family were resistant to an outside visit. In this way the student nurses were helped to realize the importance of training in group dynamics as a necessary preliminary to home visits. The role of the social worker was also clarified by a technique of this kind.

A serious rivalry problem began to appear between the nurses and the social work department, which at this time included two trained psychiatric social workers, two untrained social workers who were largely concerned with an activity programme in the hospital, a director of rehabilitation and an occupational thera- pist. This heterogeneous group was brought under the umbrella of social work to fulfil their need to have a group identity which would allow them to feel able to develop an independent role in the face of opposition from nursing, who outnumbered them significantly.

The nursing staff tended to see anyone not associated with the ward life of the patient as an interloper and a possible threat. In this context the social work department was seen as interfering with the freedom of the nurses to move out into the community and in following up ex-patients. Although an uneasy relationship was to continue during the whole period of my stay at Dingleton, the integration in the community between nurses and social workers slowly grew; but the integration in the work and activity therapy programmes was never wholly satisfactory.

The involvement of the nursing staff in decision-making on all matters concerning patient welfare was improving slowly. By the late summer of 1963 we were having serious difficulties with the top administration of the nursing hierarchy. This was made up of Matron and her deputy, both female, and two assistant matrons, both male. In my opinion, Matron and her deputy were both worthy people, well-motivated, deeply interested in the patients' welfare and skilled in psychiatry as it had been prac- tised in psychiatric hospitals up to that time. When I tried to introduce the therapeutic community concept into Dingleton they responded very positively at first, as has been described in my account of the first six months. However, as the sharing of res- ponsibility, authority and decision-making with all levels of staff and patients increased, the expectations of the role of Matron and her deputy inevitably changed. The fact that Matron had previously to take almost total responsibility for the nursing staff before my arrival made it extremely difficult for her to now sud- denly change. Moreover, two-way communication with the ex- pression of feeling meant that increasingly the senior nursing staff were put in the position of being confronted and their per- formance was discussed and criticized. This metamorphosis was

inevitably painful and was, of course, not restricted to the two
senior nurses. It affected all the senior staff of whatever discipline. The close relationship and confidence which existed
between Matron and her deputy did not extend to the two male
assistant matrons. Individually both competent people, they
nevertheless felt very insecure in the changing structure around
them.

By the end of my first year at Dingleton I was still having considerable difficulty in playing an administrative therapy role. I
was also being seen by other people as being too active and controlling. This aspect of my personality was later met by the
emergence of several alternative leaders who could 'contain' my
exuberance (Jones, 1976a, p. 34). This applied particularly to
my role relationship with my peers. By trying to play both a
supportive and interpretive role in relation to Matron, I was
tending to be seen as backing her up too much at the expense of
other staff members. In retrospect, I think it is entirely probable
that I was in too much of a hurry, even though I was well aware
of the fact that it would take a period of five years or longer to
establish some form of therapeutic community and to realize at
least some of my expectations.

Patients - the changing culture
During the second six months of my stay at Dingleton, marked
changes began to appear in the role of the patient. The change
in the authority structure for the nurses and staff generally was
accompanied by a similar change in the world of the patient. At
first there was a grave danger that greater freedom would be
mistaken for permissiveness or licence. In fact, within a therapeutic community freedom is associated with responsibility.
Abuse of freedom, if fed back to various meetings, meant that
the individuals concerned would be asked to discuss their behaviour. This concept of controls from within rather than control
from without really asks much more of the individual than does
a strict, hierarchical authority system. In my early days at
Henderson Hospital (1947-59) the patients, many of whom knew
prison well, said that the freedom in a therapeutic community
was much more demanding and painful than was the strict regime
of a prison. In prison the controls from without meant freedom
from personal responsibility, which in many ways asked less of
the individual than did the freer climate of a therapeutic community. In view of the difficulties the nursing and other staff
personnel had in adjusting to the concept of a therapeutic community, it was not surprising that patients also found themselve
confused, perplexed and, at times, angry with the new system.

In an effort to clarify the misunderstanding about appropriate
behaviour and to enable the staff and patients to come to a
shared decision about this issue, the following statement appeare
in the weekly news-sheet, published by the senior staff, of
9 July 1963, which all staff and patients received and later discussed at their ward meetings.

There seems to be some confusion among both patients and
staff about what constitutes ordinary behaviour and the
opposite. Surely we want to apply the standards of behaviour
which are accepted by the outside public and refrain from behaviour which might lead to the distress or embarrassment of
others. Patients should be given as much freedom and responsibility as they are capable of handling themselves, and
along with the staff should accept the responsibility for other
patients. This idea of teamwork is central to our thinking and
we must share our worries about ourselves and others. Thus,
concern about a patient's behaviour with the opposite sex
should be freely discussed in ward meetings or reported to the
staff in order that the supposedly offending patient's behaviour
can be discussed in his or her presence, and misunderstanding
corrected. Sometimes, because of illness, the patient's control
over his behaviour may be insufficient, and more supervision
and control from the group may be necessary. Thus, an
alcohol addict who has 'stopped' drinking may be allowed into
town with a responsible patient or nurse. But the whole ward
must lend its support and do its best to prevent the alcoholic
going off at night for a 'quick one'. Any such behaviour or
other irregular practices should be reported back to the ward
meeting or to staff personnel. This is *our* hospital and its
effectiveness in treatment and reputation in the public mind is
the responsibility of us all, both patients and staff. We want
freedom with responsible behaviour. When this is abused, we
must study the situation and try to learn from it in face-to-
face discussion. We want to help people to lead ordinary lives
and not simply discipline them; to discipline themselves rather
than to have us disciplining them; to live outside the hospital
rather than having to remain here.

The general distribution of this news-sheet was followed by an
opportunity for the whole staff to discuss its contents, and in
particular their attitude toward a more liberal regime for the
patients.
By the end of September 1963 a beginning was made to include
relatives in discussion groups with patients. At first this was
done on a very modest scale by introducing family members into
existing patient treatment groups. When patients left hospital,
this type of supportive treatment was made available through the
medium of home visits in which both nurses and social workers
participated.
The financial income of the patients was the subject of a special
study by the rehabilitation officer, Jim. Every patient in the hospital was assessed in relation to the income that he received from
any outside source, and where none was forthcoming the government grant of ten shillings a week, paid to all patients in psychiatric hospitals, was made available. In addition, as the work
therapy programme developed, a serious attempt was made to
provide appropriate amounts of pay for work done. A few of the

most successful were made group leaders with a pay ceiling of
£1 per week. By the end of the first year, the patients demonstrated in a very impressive way their capacity to run the canteen with only minimal supervision from the staff. The canteen
was becoming the social centre for the hospital and filled an
enormous gap in the life of the patients, particularly after
5.00 p.m. Rewards were now strictly in relation to patients'
performance in a work situation and this was the early beginning
of a money-incentive scheme. Relics of the custodial era, such as
a tobacco issue or 'patient orderlies' who were at the beck and
call of senior staff, were completely eliminated. We still had a
long way to go before we had anything approaching a functional
role for all the patients. Some were able to operate within a
work system. Others needed a simplified activity programme
geared to the needs of severely handicapped patients unable to
participate in any work programme. We began to experiment with
patients doing work in an outside setting. Thus, six of our
patients attended an electronics factory in a nearby town, but
they were unable to become absorbed into the social system of
the factory. This venture did not last long and probably failed
because we did not have enough emotional investment in its
success. Unlike work therapy programmes, which were then
fashionable in psychiatric hospitals in the UK, we preferred to
find work roles within the hospital structure. This was a highly
controversial issue and we were certainly in the minority in
preferring a hospital work programme to one based on outside
industry. Our general feeling was that when a patient had
reached the top of the rehabilitation ladder in the hospital, he
was then in a position to succeed in outside employment. Until
that point was reached, the emphasis was on work group therapy.
Here, difficulties in relationships with other patients, or with
staff supervisors, could be worked through and used as a learning situation. This was difficult to achieve in an industrial
setting. The fact was that, like all progressive psychiatric hospitals, we were attempting to place as many of our patients back
in the community as we possibly could. The ends were the same
but the means were somewhat different, and we were developing
our own counterculture.

Administration - the changing culture
The changing role of patients and staff inevitably implied considerable stress at the administrative level. How flexible and
open to change would the hospital administration, including the
Board of Management, prove to be? In line with our increased
emphasis on rehabilitation and functional roles for patients was
our need to economize on staff expenditure. We tried to make a
virtue out of necessity by developing work therapy or 'home
groups' where patients took over much of the housekeeping
duties previously performed by ward orderlies. Provided this
was done primarily to give the patients a functional role and not
to exploit them, this seemed to us to be a very worthwhile aim.

On 6 September 1963, I noted:

> This is the first week that we have done without the nursing
> orderlies. Personally I see this as a good thing. Reg has
> appeared as a natural leader who has been doing wonders in
> getting patients to make beds, etc., and in being much more
> active than ever previously.

The transition of Reg from a 'trouble-maker' to a creative leader
was of great importance. The issue described above would almost
certainly have found him leading the opposition had this occurred
several months previously.

During the second six months of my tenure at Dingleton, we
introduced a programme aimed at improving the patients' meal
times. At lunch patients were given an opportunity to choose a
menu for the following day. This created many problems because
patients had often forgotten what had been ordered by them the
day before, and wanted something different when the meal was
actually served! Nevertheless, the effort did help to underline
the staff's concern to raise the status of the patient. This, along
with the growing interest in the pay incentive scheme in relation
to work therapy, the establishment of a really good patient/staff
canteen, and a much more active rehabilitation programme, all
helped to raise morale.

The administration, headed by Mr Millar, had a hand in almost
every change effected during the first year, and the hospital
Board of Management which he served could not have been more
co-operative and helpful. They took a keen interest in everything
that was going on, but in no way tried to limit any efforts which
could conceivably help with patient care. The physical environment of the patients was being steadily improved, thanks to a
remarkably able architect, Mr Peter Womersley, whom we were
able to employ. Dingy geriatric wards were given much greater
window space, drapes and furniture were made bright and cheer-
ful, corridors were soundproofed, and so on. Mr Millar was
largely responsible for our early contact with the local high
school. The sixth form visited Dingleton at the end of June and
a staff team from Dingleton then had a seminar about mental
health with the same form in the school setting. This began a
growing interest between Dingleton and the schools in our
vicinity.

SUMMARY OF THE FIRST YEAR

I chose to become the superintendent of a mental hospital in
order to observe the effect that such power and authority would
have on the process of change in the direction of an open system.
Having experienced the frustrations which follow when sanctions
from higher authority are negative, I was eager to see if a traditional hospital with a characteristic hierarchical social organiz-

ation could develop a democratic egalitarian structure, if sanctions from above were positive. A model of such a kind is much
easier to accomplish with a new hospital and a staff who seek to
work in an open system. However, I thought the first priority
was to attempt such a metamorphosis in an old hospital which
reflected the characteristics of mental hospitals in general.

Initially I was imposing my ideas regarding social structure on
others, but how else can one initiate change (Jones, 1976a,
p. 25)? However, I tried to fit the methodology of social learning
that I understood and believed in to the circumstances as they
arose, for example, to resolve conflicts, rivalries, confusion,
etc., by initiating the process of interacting in a group situation
with a view to learning as a social process.

It was first necessary to familiarize myself with the social
organization of Dingleton at the time of my arrival in December
1962, which is described in stage one of this chapter. I soon became aware of a split between the senior nursing staff and the
doctors. No clear lines of authority existed, communication was
largely absent and decisions came about in a haphazard manner.
This led to the establishment of our first Senior Staff Committee
(SSC) on a bi-weekly basis, two days after my arrival. This
bringing together of hostile senior staff members was the beginning of many other regularly scheduled meetings (Jones, 1976a,
pp. 21-3), always in response to a functional need. Overtly,
such meetings had a problem-solving or administrative purpose,
but covertly they served as training situations (Jones, 1968a,
pp. 91-8), where the principles of communication theory, learning theory and systems theory could be demonstrated and role
modelled.

It proved relatively easy to establish various meetings so that
the social organization could favour this form of development.
Getting people to use the channels of communication freely at a
factual and feeling level would, I knew, take several years. At
the end of three months we had made a beginning. The Senior
Staff Committee helped me to avoid being put into the position of
having to make unilateral decisions. By indicating my wish to
discuss all matters affecting patient care and management with
my senior colleagues, the centre of power and authority was
widened to include these colleagues (the SSC). I used my
authority to establish this body, but at the same time realized
that by doing this I was initiating a change in the authority
structure to a more democratic one. Decisions shared by a group
of people inevitably involve discussion. The discussants all have
a share in the decision-making. So, from the very beginning,
the concept of decision-making by consensus was implicit in our
SSC (Jones, 1976a, pp. 57-9).

Clearly, one committee was unable to deal with all the business
and within the first three months a weekly meeting had been
established in three other areas: the Work Therapy Subcommittee
which concerned itself with patients' activities of a therapeutic
kind; the Nursing Subcommittee, which looked at the problems

concerning this particular group; and a Medical Subcommittee.
In addition, a monthly evening meeting open to all employees
of the hospital was established. Here, feelings could be expressed
which might not find an outlet in the more formal groups already
mentioned. This early attempt at creating an administrative structure which encouraged interaction around significant issues was
the beginning of a philosophy of shared decision-making and
change.

The rapid introduction of two-way communication and the
beginnings of shared decision-making within weeks of my arrival
may seem precipitate to most people and raises the whole issue of
style of leadership (Jones, 1968a, pp. 25-47). I felt that people
expected change and had a right to see my hand from the start.
I already had published two books and many articles on the
general principles of a therapeutic community, and although few
people at Dingleton had read my publications, the general principles were familiar to many of the staff. To have played a
participant-observer role and familiarize myself with the culture
of Dingleton over a longer period of time would have meant to
miss the anticipatory interest of the 'honeymoon period' which I
felt would initiate an evolutionary process.

Open communication in a democratic social organization inevitably has an equilibrating function on the system as a whole. The
fact that my authority could be questioned started a process of
listening, interacting and learning in a group setting. This process is illustrated at the beginning of this chapter (see pp. 14
and 17), when Reg, a male nurse, pointed out that the Nursing
Subcommittee had not been democratically elected. My response,
as described, was both manipulative and defensive, and showed
my own difficulty in living up to the ideal of delegating responsibility and authority to the system. Reg, by playing the role of
risk-taker, forced the administration to look at its somewhat
undemocratic behaviour (decision-making) and lack of trust
(Jones, 1976a, pp. 23-4). This is an early example of painful learning which forced me to admit my error. As the system evolved,
all representatives had to be elected democratically.

Another difficulty about having power and not abusing it
became clear in the tendency of many people, both staff and
patients, to confuse freedom with licence. I was accused of
condoning sexual relations among the patients; in an attempt to
clarify the new value system a statement from the hospital
administration appeared in the weekly 'News-sheet'. The clash
between the old (moral) order and the new open-system approach
was reflected by the conflict of values between two of the doctors.
The fact that I had 'shown interest in the attractive laundry
supervisor' only reinforced my image as an amoral person in the
conservative culture in this part of Scotland. This image was to
cause problems throughout my entire seven years at Dingleton
and is almost a predictable process when a male leader advocates
changing the culture of a hospital from a closed to an open
system. Freedom to many people seems to imply sexual freedom.

Within two months, many of the principles of an open system were being discussed and either adopted or modified by group discussion; in the process I was learning. A climate for change was already present in the hospital, thanks to the leadership of Dr Ken Morrice. Usually the top establishment resists change either overtly or covertly and in this sense we were off to a flying start. This meant that to some extent other people were identified with the task of evolving a therapeutic community, and it was no longer 'my' project. During the initial two-month period parallel developments were occurring in the upper echelons of the hospital, that is, in the Board of Management and in various hospital subgroups.

I knew that the role I chose to play clinically would be important. Within weeks I was assuming clinical responsibility for some interviews with new patients and inviting other staff members to be present to establish a new pattern of shared responsibility and interest with the line staff. But the main thrust was to evolve a social structure with a heavy emphasis on function. Social structure and function form two dimensions in any theory of social systems (Parsons, 1960). In the narrower sense of the term, 'social structure' refers to a system of differentiated roles, how they are distributed within the social system, and how they are integrated with each other. 'Social system' is concerned with interaction between individuals involved in the interactional process which is the essential part of a social system. In this context, a role concerns itself with the quality of relationships which the individual forms with others and the functional significance that this has for the social system. In social systems theory, function concerns itself with the dynamics of motivational processes, such as the maintenance of stability or production of change, or the integration or disruption of the social system.

How could patients and staff use the time available most effectively to interact, listen and learn? It was in this context that meetings mushroomed, but always with a clear purpose and tangible outcome. If 'nothing happened' at such meetings (an uncommon occurrence), then we learned to assume that the failure was ours and a solution must be sought. Was it lack of skill in agenda building; or 'prima donnas' dominating the meeting, abusing their power, failing to listen to other inputs, etc.? In other words, we were learning about the learning process. Despite such good intentions some meetings failed in their purpose and after weeks or months would be discontinued. The important issue at this early stage of our development was to demonstrate that if meetings were boring (to some) and could not effect change, then there was no point in meetings for meetings' sake. The number, composition, time-span and identity of the meetings (work therapy, night nurses, etc.) was a measure of our skill in organization, flexibility and willingness to learn by trial and error.

The 'honeymoon phase' lasted approximately two months, and when the reaction occurred, it came from the relatively junior

nursing staff. They criticized their lack of involvement in planning, overlooking the fact that Matron was their representative
at all meetings of the Senior Staff Committee which was meeting
twice a week. However, it seemed clear that feedback and feed
forward throughout the nursing system was at an embryonic
stage (Jones, 1968a, pp. 54-7). This led to an attempt to integrate both ends of the nursing spectrum in a regularly scheduled
nursing meeting, open to all nurses, so that interaction and
social learning became possible. We, the administration, could
learn from the system just as could everyone else.

From the start I tried to avoid the trap of making unilateral
decisions. As already mentioned, within two days of my arrival
the Senior Staff Committee - comprising twelve senior people,
leaders in the various divisions of the hospital both clinical and
administrative - was formed, and all decisions were funnelled
through this committee. In this way the concept of shared
decision-making was established (Jones, 1968a, pp. 48-67), and
unilateral decisions became virtually impossible.

We also began planning meetings with the local authority
Medical Officers of Health representing the four Border counties.
We discussed our overlapping roles in promoting health care, and
the need to integrate with the 68 family doctors in our catchment
area. Home visits to prospective patients, accompanied by the
family doctor, were initiated about this time.

During the second half of the first year, the resistances to
change, which had no doubt been present all along, now became
more overt. In particular, the doctors and senior nursing staff
were beginning to feel threatened by the growing tendency to be
questioned by junior staff about their role performance. This
was an inevitable by-product of opening up communication
throughout the hospital system. Meetings were becoming less
inhibited, and junior staff no longer remained silent while 'listening' to their seniors. Fear of reprisal was disappearing as any
threats of this kind could be fed back to the following meeting.
In other words the abuse of authority was 'contained' (Jones,
1976a, pp. 34-5). All this meant a change in everyone's perception of his/her role and this applied most to those people with
the greatest authority, for example, Matron, brought up in
traditional hospital practice where her word was law in the nursing sphere, now had to avoid making unilateral decisions or face
discussion of her behaviour from her peers or even from junior
nurses. To some degree also, her perception of her role had to
conform to the role deemed most appropriate by the system as a
whole. Sometimes her self-control broke down and she 'regressed'
to the old authoritarian role by angrily crushing her 'tormentors'.
But she always regretted these lapses and we were able to use
such episodes as a learning experience for everyone.

I felt considerable guilt in the conflict that was inevitable in
Matron's attempt to modify her role in conforming to the expectations of an open system. This empathy and my gratitude to her
for her willingness to try combined to make me spend many hours

in her office, often talking late into the night. It was a sort of combination teacher-therapist-pupil role and was a corrective influence for me. As a result I became aware of the rather repressive Catholic culture for which she was the rallying point for a significant part of the hospital population. But for her corrective influence as the representative of the old culture, I might have made some disastrous mistakes.

Although Dr Small also represented a rallying point for the 'old guard', she was barely on speaking terms with Matron so that the opposition to the process of change had two totally different leaders. Whereas Matron was willing to change despite the anguish it caused her, Dr Small retained her disapproval and in that sense was a serious negative factor in the system. Even so, she steadily lost ground as more people were affected by the learning process and after her retirement three years later no one emerged to take her place as the opposition leader.

Despite all the difficulites, the role of the patient was changing steadily (Jones, 1968a, pp. 60-6), and the role relationship between patients and nurses was far more egalitarian than previously. Patients were playing more functional roles and the idea of pay for work done was beginning to attract attention. Part of this evolution was the increasing delegation of responsibility and authority throughout the system, and this included patients as well as staff. By the end of the first year they had their own canteen run largely by patient staff, their own monthly magazine and their relatives were encouraged to attend treatment groups.

Finally, the physical environment of the patients was changing dramatically thanks to an outstanding architect. He was engaged by the Board of Management, who saw their main function as that of helping the staff to realize every goal that was aimed at improving the patients' welfare - a unique phenomenon in my experience!

Chapter 2

The second year, 1964:
problems of leadership and consensus

INTRODUCTION

Our aim in the second year was to consolidate the gains in open
communication and shared decision-making which had made considerable progress during the first twelve months. However, the
trust level was not yet very high and this pertained particularly
to the nursing staff (Jones, 1976a, pp. 23-4). The more junior
levels felt themselves to be relatively uninvolved in planning in
issues which involved them directly. Although Matron represented their interests at the Senior Staff Committee, etc., they
were not consulted beforehand so that, in fact, she was assuming
that she understood their views without having actually discussed matters with them. On the positive side was the fact that
criticism from junior nurses was becoming more overt and Matron
was beginning to accept this change in the quality of her role
relationship with them.

Other stresses were appearing as a result of the beginning of
the transition from a closed to a more open system. A few of us
with previous experience of this approach were prepared for
more painful communication as we became more exposed to
rumours and other misunderstandings which in a less open culture might have remained largely covert.

MONTHS TWELVE TO EIGHTEEN

Nursing
During this period the senior nursing staff became much more
a part of the hospital than had been the case during the first
year. The senior nurses were the same as before, but seemed to
have less conflict with the medical staff and with other staff
members than previously. This, I think, was partly due to the
skills of the new assistant matrons who had been recruited.
Instead of two assistant matrons, one for the male and one for
the female side, we now had three assistant matrons (two men
and one woman), all identified with the hospital as a whole, plus
a male nurse tutor. Two of the new assistants were very active
and articulate young men who, though not afraid of original
thought, fully understood the intricacies of the nursing profession and the need to respect much of its conservatism. In
keeping with this positive growth was a much greater willingness
to bring about change and to initiate change. For example, I

noted in my diary on 14 March 1964:

> Undoubtedly the great event of the week has been the completio
> on Thursday of the document, 'Proposed reorganization of
> ward staffing'. This is a triumph for the nursing staff, and in
> particular their handling of the Matron in getting the whole
> plan for a three-shift (eight-hour) system through. We are
> now going to have an open meeting of the nursing staff on
> Monday to see how they react to this proposed plan. Although
> the nurses, in the first instance, expressed a great eagerness
> to have an eight-hour day, when it comes to actually facing
> change it seems they are not so keen. In fact, there has been
> a splinter group who have been trying to organize all the
> nurses into protesting any change and who wish to remain on
> a twelve-hour day. I think it is probable that this is no more
> than the usual resistance to change and that this splinter
> group should not be taken too seriously. Anyway, we will
> know on Monday.
> The great advantage of the new plan is that it should leave
> the nurses much fresher for their work with the patients,
> and it should make recruitment easier. The possible young
> recruit dreads the prospect of working twelve hours at a
> stretch. The plan also allows for an overlap between the
> morning and evening shifts of one hour, and the same thing
> at night, so that the night staff are less cut off from the day
> staff. In addition, there will be more nurses in the evening to
> organize and participate in patient activities. Matron could
> never have drawn up this plan on her own, and the slow
> development of the senior nursing group as an extension of
> herself has been immensely effective. She is no longer the only
> power figure for our nurses, and I think that she is beginning
> to appreciate that this gives her a positive image she never
> had when she dealt with things alone. Surrounded by her
> satellites she can now avoid answering questions which she is
> not sure about, and knows that one of her bright assistants
> will answer it for her. If she disagrees with what one of them
> says she can immediately jump on him/her, but if she approves
> she can bask in the illusion that all the ideas really come from
> her. We now have a fairly adequate nursing establishment and
> hope to be able to put the three-shift day into operation with
> our existing staff. We fall short of our actual required estab-
> lishment by one charge nurse, four staff nurses and from
> ten to twenty student or pupil nurses. [Student nurses at this
> time did a three-year training to qualify as Registered Mental
> Nurses, and pupil nurses did a two-year training as Assistant
> Nurses.]

This is not to imply that the assistant matrons necessarily agreed
with their two senior colleagues. The real change was in their
capacity to implement whatever ideas were developed.
  It is, I think, important to note that during the first year it

was Matron and her deputy who appeared to provide the greatest
resistance to change. In retrospect I do not see this as all negative. On the contrary, I am indebted to Matron for preventing
the catastrophe which might well have followed too rapid a rate
of change in a hospital which had become quite set in its ways.
The staff lived and had in most cases grown up in the neighbourhood. They were part of a local community of a conservative
kind. Matron had a braking effect on my tendency of over-
enthusiasm and exuberance. I could sometimes convince myself
and other people that a new idea would work before it had been
fully digested. With the advent of the second year and a much
stronger senior nursing staff there was much more security at
the top of the nursing hierarchy. This meant a greater capacity
to deal with the anxieties which change caused in the lower
echelons of nursing as well as in other parts of the staff structure.

The leadership in nursing was becoming dynamic but we still
had a long way to go before this change was apparent at all
levels of the nursing hierarchy. As an example of this one can
cite the fate of the 'Grand Plan'. An immense amount of work
went into this reorganization of the hospital nursing body so
that the nurses could work an eight-hour instead of a twelve-
hour day. The minutes of the Senior Staff Committee were largely
concerned with this topic at every meeting between 17 February
and May 1964. At the open meeting with the nursing staff held
on 16 March the majority favoured a three-shift system, but did
not like the one that had been presented to them as a working
model by the senior nurses. It was suggested that they produce
their own plan and a second meeting was arranged for two weeks
later. At this meeting the junior nurses' plan was adopted by an
overwhelming majority. It seemed that some of the nursing staff
were hostile toward the 'management' and wanted to put them
down by developing their own plan. By 6 April the minutes of
the Senior Staff Committee recorded:

On the subject of the three-shift system the Matron doubted
if the plan presented by the junior nurses could be implemented
with the present nursing numbers and with nurses off sick,
etc. The assistant matrons also felt that the present staffing
position made the plan impossible. However, the Matron said
she would try to draw up a plan, using available personnel, to
see how this came out on paper. Although it appeared that the
majority of the nursing staff wanted their own plan for a three-
shift system, it was thought that there were still some staff
who wanted to keep the 'long day of twelve hours'. Jimmy
Millar wondered if nursing staff were telling the management
what hours they wanted to work without due regard for the
good of the patients. Dr Ken Morrice thought that we were in a
very difficult situation. If we did not implement the junior
nurses' plan, nursing staff would say that the senior staff
never tried to do what *they* wanted. He did not think we should

be too hasty about implementing the plan. The SSC members felt that although Dr Jones seemed to think we must try to give the nursing staff the system they wanted, the SSC had not committed themselves; a clear indication that the medical superintendent could be overruled and that we were already committed to group decision-making. Care would have to be taken that we did not inaugurate a system which senior staff and nurses later regretted. Dr Morrice said that although we were disappointed at staff reaction to the original senior nurses' plan, there was a large body of nursing staff who genuinely felt they were being pushed around and had to fall in with what the SSC wanted, thus indicating a trend to extend shared decision-making beyond the SSC and involve the junior levels of staff as well.

The minutes of the Senior Staff Committee of 9 April 1964 stated:

Regarding the three-shift system there was considerable discussion as to whether or not this could be implemented, even if the majority of staff really wanted it. It was not clear if they actually preferred the present long day with compensating time off on several consecutive days. The Matron said that the latter seemed to suit best the married women with home commitments. Nurse Drummond felt there was a body of staff who would go either way. Dr Small thought the shortage of nurses was causing a great deal of anxiety to staff, but it was pointed out that the nurses must know that we were well aware of this, and were doing all we could to recruit new staff. It was felt whatever plan was evolved, it must be the best plan for the care of the patients. Also, if any shift system was put into operation, it would have to be made clear that it was an experimental plan, subject to modification, and would be for a trial-and-error period of two or three months only and then reviewed. Decisions about hospital policy could not be made merely because the majority favoured a certain position. We still had responsibilities to patients and the community outside. It should also be made clear that although a great deal of authority was being delegated to junior staff, we [the SSC] must retain the right to veto anything which we felt to be detrimental to the ultimate good of the hospital.

In retrospect, it seems to me that this is a good example of a decision-making process which failed to achieve consensus (Jones, 1968a, pp. 48-67). Reading all the available documents I am left with the opinion that although the senior staff had a certain amount of awareness of the problem from their point of view and did considerable 'homework' in preparing various draft designs, they were not fully in touch with the feeling among the nurses generally. As an example of this, the night nurses were never really involved in the whole process of dis-

cussion. Staff were split into different subgroups not only on the basis of status, but by other factors, such as part-time outside employment and so on. No one nursing attitude emerged, and while the senior staff could plan something that would be ideal for patients' 24-hour care, teaching and so on, they were not themselves going to be affected by the plan which was pre-dominantly in relation to the positions of charge nurses down-ward. The junior ranks of the nursing profession showed no evidence of leadership among their peers, and so after two months of frequent meetings a stalemate resulted. One could say that the plan simply withered. Had the more junior nurses had a deep investment in an eight-hour day they could have easily revived the whole issue. As it was they seemed to be con-tent to accept the Matron's decision that our present nursing personnel were not sufficiently numerous to put such a plan into action. It is worth mentioning that the eight-hour day was never achieved in my time as superintendent, but came later when sufficient nurses were available. This attempt at shared decision-making shows our relatively immature stage of evolution to an open system at that time. Communication of content and feeling, information-sharing and feedback were incomplete, but some social learning was, I think, achieved (Jones, 1968a, pp.68-107).

The increased confidence at the top of the nursing hierarchy was reflected in improved recruitment and improved teaching. The nurse tutor had able assistance from the three young assist-ant matrons. In collaboration with first the Matron, and then Michael Clark, one of the new assistant matrons, two articles de-scribing therapeutic community principles appeared in the nursing journals (Jones and Mullen, 1963; Jones and Clark, 1965).

It was at this time the planning of a one-year post-registration course in psychiatry for nurses who had completed their general nurse training was started. Many hospitals did an eighteen-month training for psychiatry, but we were given to understand that we might be the first hospital in Scotland which would be allowed to attempt a one-year training of this kind.

Better recruitment at all levels acted like a transfusion to the nursing body. People began to realize that holding a nursing job was not simply a matter of conforming, and advancement in their professional career became increasingly competitive. The staff nurses who were on the staff when I arrived felt that job-advancement opportunities were too scarce. Instead of automatic promotion they were now told by the SSC in no uncertain fashion that it was not a question of filling dead men's shoes, and that if they were enterprising and sought experience elsewhere their chances of promotion on returning to Dingleton would be improved.

Patients

Along with the improvement in nursing morale, the patients were given every encouragement to become more independent and active. The daily groups in each of the wards were complemented by the start of family groups, where two or more families met

together under staff supervision. A series of new patients with
severe character disorders caused considerable concern in the
hospital and its surrounds. As a result of the anxiety generated,
a growing interest emerged in studying the dynamics of behaviour
and coming to some understanding of what caused a disturbance.
The analysis of behaviour involved patients as much as staff in
both formal and informal group situations (Jones, 1968a, pp.
42-7). The responsibility patients had for one another and how
far they helped in the treatment programme became more
explicit. It was about this time that we began to talk about the
possible division of the hospital into three county teams, representing the county areas which we served, although actual
decentralization was still some time away.

One interesting effect of the better social conditions for
patients, particularly the new social centre and canteen, was
that they went out of the hospital much less frequently than
previously. It was commented by people in Melrose that they
saw our patients hardly at all. There had been some feeling that
we might be depriving local tradesmen of patient trade but this
never amounted to anything much. At that time our goal of
community involvement for patients was still barely conceptualized. But we certainly did not want to insulate them from the
community at large, and patients were free to come and go as
they chose as part of the open-door policy. Nevertheless, the
patient/staff canteen continued to thrive and the profits were
quite considerable. We began to discuss how the profit could be
returned to the patients for things which they felt would aid
their own rehabilitation, but nothing definite was established.
We began to talk about a patients' 'pub' in addition to the canteen, but this met with a surprising amount of disapproval from
the patients themselves and was never implemented.

Physicians on the medical staff
During this period - twelve to eighteen months after my arrival
at Dingleton - we still had, in order of seniority, two consultants,
one senior hospital medical officer, one registrar and one senior
house officer. We were acutely conscious of the fact that if we
were to develop, particularly in community work, we would need
a more numerous medical staff. We put pressure on the Regional
Board and got a good deal of response, because an extension of
our staff had already been recommended by an official report to
Scottish hospitals. It was at this time, too, that I suggested to
my colleague, Dr Ken Morrice, that he might like to do an exchange for a year with one of the doctors whom I knew at Fort
Logan Mental Health Center in Denver, Colorado. Ken liked the
idea and realized that it would be a valuable training experience
for him. During this period the only addition to our staff was a
part-time senior house officer who helped in the geriatric wards.
She was married to a local minister and proved a very real help
in this rather neglected area of our practice.

We were already attracting many prominent visitors from the

USA and Europe, but unfortunately rather fewer from the UK.
This cross-fertilization helped us to have a holistic view of
mental health at that time. A well-known professor from the US
said that if we had paid as much attention to individual treatment as we did to group treatment, then we would have a model
as good as, if not better than, anything in psychiatry at the
present time. He suggested that for this advance we should
have a relationship with Edinburgh Medical School much like that
which Topeka State Hospital had with the University of Kansas.
He felt that our attraction for American psychiatrists was greater
than that of British universities, and that it would be to the
advantage of the university to sponsor our efforts. It is only
fair to say that all along the leaders of the department of psychiatry in Edinburgh had been most helpful, and involved us in
their teaching programme. The American professor said that we
were criticized mostly because our therapeutic community practice
put the emphasis on the process rather than on the outcome.
This is a true statement to the present day. At the same time
we had made every effort to obtain research money so that we
could pay much more attention to results, but we received only
limited help from research grants. One might add that if the
process is correct, a positive and successful outcome is assured;
it simply follows naturally.

About this time my relationship with my deputy, Dr Ken
Morrice, became more strained. To quote from my 'Impressions'
dated 1 February 1964:

It seems that there is a possible danger of a staff split and I
shall attempt to analyse this. The female hospital ward has a
small, integrated and articulate group led by Dr Ken Morrice.
He is, of course, my deputy and by and large seems to be
identified with the goals of a therapeutic community. At the
same time he acts as an autonomous head of the female side and
is particularly close to two senior nurses and Dr Small. Those
four people tend to be rather exclusive and operate entirely
from their own territory and have not very much identification
with the hospital as a whole. Dr Morrice manages to keep on
pretty good terms with me, although he must feel considerable
conflict at times. I think he deals with these feelings by pro-
jecting them on to the male side of the hospital run by Dr
Ratcliffe. Thus, if we take an example: a male patient, Eric,
represents a very serious management problem and is a potentially dangerous patient. If Dr Small is on duty over the weekend
she may have to deal with this patient and she is understandably terrified. Her fears extend to her living quarters which
are open to the outside public. She feels the need for greater
control of the male patients, and to her this means through
physical treatment generally, including ECT and tranquillizers.
Dr Small has a great capacity to arouse people's anxieties and
can get a ready response from the female hospital group, particularly as her anxieties usually refer to the male side and

there is an understandable ready-made rivalry situation between the two sides. The male side, on the other hand, has
no such closely knit system. Dr Ratcliffe operates in a much
more independent way and demands no particular loyalties
from his staff. Dr Mair, his assistant, is at the opposite pole
from Dr Small and, if anything, generates too little anxiety,
and is inclined to let dangerous situations develop. This, of
course, arouses Dr Small's anxiety which is communicated to
her senior, Dr Ken Morrice. Dr Mair is a disciple of mine, but
carries my ideas further than I would.

I have been fairly intimately concerned with this patient,
Eric, and feel that Dr Ratcliffe has a pretty good grasp of the
dynamic factors involved, including the whole family constel-
lation. Dr Ratcliffe knows what he is doing and why he is doing
it. At the same time, the threat of violence is there. This sets
off the anxieties of the female wards which ultimately, as I see
it, results in a rather absurd situation where Dr Morrice, responding to these anxieties and yet knowing very little about
the details of the case, expresses his belief that Eric is being
wrongly treated and should be given ECT.

There is a sort of middle group which includes the social
workers and, to some extent, the nursing administration who
are not identified with either side of the hospital. As they are
not intimately concerned with the physical management of Eric,
they are not responding to any personal feelings of danger.
This middle group is, I think, asserting a constant and modify-
ing educational influence on the hospital as a whole. In addition
there is Dr Morrice's own interest in psychiatry and his preference for psychotherapy when it can be used effectively, but
he accepts the necessity for physical treatment in appropriate
cases. He supplies a constant corrective experience to Dr
Small's excesses.

On Wednesday, quite impulsively, I gave Dr Morrice my above
'Impressions' for 1 February to read. It seemed to me this was
an interesting and honest, if somewhat daring, experiment.
Clearly I had had no such intention when I had written them,
but I thought it might be easier to get my meaning through to
Dr Morrice by the written rather than the spoken word. He
replied in writing as follows:

Re yours 'Impressions', 1 February 1964 - following my outspoken comments of this morning [2 February 1964], there is
probably little to add.

On the whole I agree with your overall perception of the situation; but I see the persistence of notions which I do not think
are very true and feel are largely irrelevant to Eric's case.

Consciously, I have no rivalry feelings vis-à-vis the Super-
intendency. Mostly, I am very glad *not* to be Medical Superintendent, and while unconscious ideas of this kind may well
exist, I am identified very closely with you. I am *not* the Crown

Prince lusting after your throne. Rather I am your Chancellor, concerned occasionally about the method of distribution of resources and - perhaps because I have been around longer - prone to hear from many quarters, feelings and resentments that are never expressed directly to you.

As I said at yesterday's SSC meeting, and as you indicate in your 'Impressions', I feel that psychiatry at present cannot afford to ignore *any* method of treatment. By the same token, in the present state of development (? undevelopment) of our culture at Dingleton, I think it folly to try to treat a very difficult, aggressive and dangerous man in a way which is sure to quickly exhaust the small resources of our staff and imperil our already tricky relationship with the community.

If this was worth trying (which I doubt) it needed a full discussion of clinical staff and some sort of agreement and a greater measure of safeguard. I do not feel nearly as satisfied as you that Dr Ratcliffe 'knows what he is doing and why he is doing it'.

I cite Malcolm and Tom as other examples of 'asking for trouble'. I think you exaggerate the split and rivalry between male and female sides. It may even be that you encourage it by pointing it out in various ways! The differences you high-light are true, but they are not the only ones. There are practical differences which are just as important as any subtle theoretical ones - I know you agree - and one cuts one's coat according to the cloth. This is what pleases and reassures me about your approach. It is realistic and unambiguous and logical. You employ sanctions where necessary. But, perhaps because you carry a great burden of responsibility and act as a support and encouragement to so many staff members, you may be tempted to see gold where there is only a buttercup!

I am after all a canny Aberdonian. It would be out of charac-ter for me to risk the hospital for the sake of one patient. Dr Ratcliffe is cannier than I *and* more anxious *and* more self-seeking. (Make what sibling rivalry interpretations you like!) So why does he take the risks? Working with him for some years now I know his good points and his bad. You have brought out more of the former into the light of day in the past year! I even recognize some of my failings - impatience, short-circuit reactions, evangelical zeal, and an eccentric wish to be normal, and - apart from the latter - I think I'm improving. But don't overestimate us.

This is part of the 'evolution of psychiatry in Scotland', and it may be slower than we want. We need a Registrar and a few brighter nurses - as well as a better social set-up (I know, they're coming). But you can't really treat patients today with tomorrow's resources. I'm with you, but give me room!

P.S.: These are hastily written notes and not to be con-sidered weightily.

Dr Morrice's statement was, I think, very fair and there was a

lot of wisdom in what he said. In retrospect one wonders why
this letter was not read to the SSC to form the basis for a living-
learning situation. We apparently were still far short of our later
practice of turning all serious conflicts into social-learning experiences.

The case of Eric was valuable in highlighting the difficulties
imposed upon us with an open-door hospital, plus a therapeutic
community approach in a setting where the peer-patient group
was still relatively weak, and where the nurses were relatively
untrained. One of the anomalies of the situation was the way in
which Dr Small reacted to her own anxiety, turning to Dr Morrice
rather than opening the whole question up for the SSC or Nursing Subcommittee to examine. It is well known that staff splits
are reflected in patient disorganization and irresponsibility
(Stanton and Swartz, 1954). The establishment of clinical meetings at times of stress was an attempt to meet this threat of
splitting the hospital into factions. We tried to act as a co-
ordinated whole when faced by a problem which affected us all
in varying degrees. At such times we needed a concerted and
co-ordinated policy so that the danger of splitting was avoided.
How far Dr Small could have co-operated in this kind of approach
remained to be seen.

Social work
At this phase in our development there were distinct signs of
growth in our outside commitments. During this period we
acquired a hospital car, primarily for use by the social workers
who might not have their own transport. The district (public
health) nurses in the Border counties were visiting Dingleton
in order to become familiar with the staff with a view to improving communications between the hospital and the outside community. We now had a young American social worker, Marcia
Jones, with a master's degree; a part-time social worker with
her British qualification of Psychiatric Social Worker (PSW);
and two unqualified social workers who were helping with patient
activities and so on. We had been working with the local authorities with a view to persuading them to employ a social worker
for themselves. In April 1964 we heard that the authorities in
Roxburghshire, Selkirkshire and Berwickshire had agreed to
pay for a PSW who would be based at Dingleton and supplied
with a house in the neighbourhood by the local authority. This
was of obvious significance in forging a link between ourselves
and the local authorities.

By now pupils and teachers from six different schools had
visited Dingleton to get a better understanding of what goes on
in a psychiatric hospital. We were also becoming increasingly
close to many of the family doctors. However, along with all these
positive trends we were becoming more aware of a growing negative image of Dingleton in the outside community. This seemed
inevitable in view of the fact that we were pushing a rehabilitation programme which meant a far more active programme for

patients and less use of chemical and other restraints. The groups
inevitably led to rumours that there was no privacy or confidentiality at Dingleton, and many people, including some family
doctors, were genuinely unhappy about our treatment approach
- it was unfamiliar and suspect in a conservative culture like
the Border country.

MONTHS EIGHTEEN TO TWENTY-FOUR:
LIVING-LEARNING SITUATIONS

During this period, eighteen to twenty-four months after my
arrival, my 'Impressions' contained much more evidence of learning as a social process or what at the time we termed living-
learning situations (Jones, 1968a, pp. 68-107; 1976a, pp. 43-53).
At this comparatively early stage of our development there was
not necessarily much skill or understanding of the methodology
associated with such a procedure. The trained staff were getting
much more interested in using situations of stress as a learning
experience. I noted:

> At the staff nurses' meeting on Thursday I was faced by a
> formidable array of staff nurses, including Reg Elliott, I had a
> visitor with me and asked if it would be alright for one or two
> visitors to join the group. They agreed somewhat grudgingly
> and it was clear that there was something on their minds.
> They immediately launched into a tirade about the way in
> which a student nurse, Alex, had been misused by Dr Ratcliffe
> and by the assistant matron, Michael Clark. Apparently a
> patient called Ned, a young schizophrenic in a very disturbed
> state, has been on large doses of largactil and had been falling
> out of bed, etc. He came into the adolescent group on Monday
> at 9.30, and had to be taken out almost immediately because he
> was falling on the floor and making the group process quite
> impossible. He then attended Dr Ratcliffe's adult group at
> 10.30 and again had to be removed because of his behaviour.
> Around lunch-time, Alex, the student nurse who had been
> looking after him a good part of the last few days, was alone
> with him and he seemed to be slipping into unconsciousness.
> Alex slapped his face and Marcia Jones, the psychiatric social
> worker, happened to be passing at the time. She was rather
> surprised at this picture and spoke to Dr Ratcliffe about it.
> He seemed to have been somewhat perturbed because the
> patient's parents were due to visit that afternoon. He spoke to
> the assistant matron who then told Alex that he was perhaps
> foolish to use this kind of stimulation in a public ward. The
> student nurse saw this as a severe reprimand which, of
> course, it was not, and apparently was very upset. He venti-
> lated his grievance and this aroused the opposition of the
> staff nurses and led to the unfriendly climate at the beginning
> of their weekly meeting which Alex had been asked to attend.

We felt that the best thing to do was to create a living-learning situation, but learned from Alex that he had already been the centre of a living-learning situation on the ward built around the incident.

It seems that Dr Ratcliffe had explained to the student nurse that the patient was suffering from toxic side-effects of the largactil and was having muscle spasms. The situation had been looked at in terms of the student's own feelings of anxiety and the uncertainty of his role. However, Alex did not feed back to the staff nurses what he had learned from this interaction with Dr Ratcliffe and was still angry and resentful. We tried to work out the reason for this tension, and it became apparent that there were two major themes. One was that the student is one of a group of disgruntled young male nurses who feel that they are being neglected, and that their teaching is not really preparing them for their nursing exams. They want to be spoon-fed as they have been in the past and resent the new kind of training based on group dynamics and living-learning situations, which they feel is not what they want to get through their exams. Alex admitted that he was feeling resentful along with these other young men and that this formed a background to his current upset. Moreover, he felt doubtful about Dr Ratcliffe's handling of the case and resented being left alone with a patient who, it seemed to him, was getting steadily worse, when he had no idea of how to handle the situation clinically. He also said that he was angry with the PSW, Marcia, for going to Dr Ratcliffe rather than talking to the nurses. Marcia, who was also in attendance, tried to explain her behaviour, rather ineffectively I thought, and said that she had not meant to cause any trouble and had really meant to talk to the nurses herself but happened to see Dr Ratcliffe first.

The other general theme then became clear: that the nurses generally feel that the social workers are privileged but 'non-clinical' personnel who may misunderstand their behaviour in their nursing role. The staff nurses said this could easily happen again and comments, such as 'the PSWs might jeopardize their jobs', were made. At a deeper level I feel pretty certain that the staff nurses see the social workers as being not only closer to the doctors, but socially more acceptable to them. The nurses feel they are at a disadvantage and in a lower-status position.

It was agreed that the student nurse had done a perfectly understandable thing in slapping this boy's face in order to test his contact with reality, and that this was a common procedure in insulin-coma treatment and so on. At the same time the PSW, Marcia, unfamiliar with ward treatment, would see this as very strange behaviour. She would understandably wonder what was going on, and find it easier to talk to Dr Ratcliffe than to the ward staff.

This really was the crux of the situation - that the social

workers relate to the doctors rather than to the nurses. I do
not think the tension was entirely relieved by the meeting, but
it certainly gave everyone a good deal of food for thought and
was a situation in which I think the senior staff were probably
wrong. The PSW, Marcia, handled the situation badly, and was
slippery and apologetic and did not sound quite truthful. Dr
Ratcliffe seems to have been over-anxious and to have acted
rather precipitously. Finally, we have learned that if Marcia
had dealt with the situation by having a meeting on the spot
with the people concerned, much misunderstanding might have
been avoided and the situation might not have escalated. But
a living-learning situation involving everyone would still have
been necessary to work through the social workers' privileged
position with the doctors.

Living-learning situations and confrontation may of course be
extremely painful (Jones, 1976a, pp. 42-3). This applies particularly to people in more senior and established positions, who
are invited to discard their protection from criticism and examination which authority usually implies. An example of this
occurred in December:

On Thursday, Nurse Reg Elliott came to the '8.30'. [The senior
administrator's meeting which was daily and met from 8.30 to
9.00 a.m., and was attended by Matron; the Hospital Secretary,
Jimmy Millar; and myself - and sometimes other senior staff.
It dealt with administrative as opposed to clinical matters.
Anyone with a grievance was welcome to attend and be heard.]
Reg complained about having been put on night duty without
being consulted. He had just come off night shift four months
ago and felt that other people should have been asked to take
their turn on this occasion. His wife was upset about his going
on night duty at such short notice, and could not understand
why he was being singled out. When Reg had finished speaking
the Matron sailed into him in a very angry way and we were
appalled to see the phenomenon of someone coming to the '8.30'
for help and then being roundly abused.
  I did my best to pour oil on troubled waters, but no one else
seemed able to take an active part. The Matron said that she
had not the slightest intention of leaving Reg on night duty
for more than the two weeks after he had come back from his
one week's leave, and that she had no alternative as things
were. Reg was very disgruntled, and asked to see me later in
the day. I saw him with an assistant matron and it seemed that
the latter was very identified with Reg's problem, and was
probably feeling very guilty because he had done nothing to
support him in the earlier meeting. Reg talked about victim-
ization and had told other people that by seeking help from the
'8.30' he had got shouted at for his trouble. Other people said,
'Well, that's what we expected', and Reg said that no one
would now use the '8.30' because of the danger of reprisals.

We tried to point out to him that there was a strong likelihood that the Matron was probably aware of her mistake and was wishing that she could modify her behaviour on occasions like this. We felt that people should continue using the '8.30' until it became a familiar pattern, and hopefully the Matron would learn to use it more effectively.

On Friday morning the Matron arrived ten minutes early for the '8.30' meeting, and said that she realized that she had been in error the previous day and wished she had not lost her temper with Reg. She talked about her own particular antipathy to him as a person, and admitted that it was a great pity that the '8.30' was seen as a place where one might meet with anger instead of understanding. I admired her very much for her honesty and we continued discussing the whole question of the use of the '8.30'. When the others came there was a general agreement that any staff member with a complaint was free to use the '8.30', and there must be no later reprisals. I was immensely impressed by the Matron's courage in admitting her own failure, and that Reg had contributed to a learning experience. I took pains to feed this back to Reg later in the day, and I think he was somewhat mollified.

It may be that I acted rather arbitrarily in seeing Reg and the senior nurse without the presence of Matron, but knowing her temperament and pride I presumably felt that she needed time to compose herself, and the facts bear this out. Confrontation is discussed frequently in this book and there may have been a tendency to stereotype procedures, thus overlooking the need for different strategies with differing personalities.

The nature and rate of change occurring at Dingleton at this time must have had an influence on most, if not all, people in the hospital then. People who had been at Dingleton before my arrival had by far the most difficult time because they had to change from an established culture to a largely new one which was constantly changing. Staff who had come to Dingleton after my arrival knew what to expect and were motivated toward therapeutic community principles. For someone at the top of the nursing hierarchy who had been at Dingleton many years before my time, the situation was fraught with difficulty. In September I noted:

The Matron seems to be reaching the limit beyond which she is not prepared to go. According to Michael Clark, an assistant matron, she feels she can go no further and that if she becomes more deviant than she now is, she will be dropped by her own peer group of hospital matrons. This prospect, he thinks, terrifies her, particularly in terms of her retirement.

It seems that my aspiration that she should retire in a blaze of glory and be seen as a pioneer is very unrealistic. She is much more concerned with the danger of being seen as something of a leper. This fits in with her behaviour this week

when she started off in the Monday night meeting by digging
in her heels and contradicting every communication I made
that had any suggestion of change. Another straw in the wind
is the fact that the Matron has shown a tendency to avoid the
'8.30' senior staff meetings whenever possible. This is quite a
new departure and reflects her desire to avoid situations which
may be challenging and may initiate change.

Despite the above, my relationship with the Matron was tending to improve, and her attitude toward therapeutic communities
was becoming more positive. By the end of 1964 I was still preoccupied with the problem of leadership and noted:

I have been at Dingleton for just over two years. The old problem of Number One and Number Two still remains, and my
relationship with Dr Morrice is still a problem, whereas the
problem with the Matron tends slowly to lessen. As far as Dr
Morrice is concerned the question of my enthusiasm is important. This concept was stressed by Norm Bell, a sociologist
from the US, when he visited last week. I tend by my enthusiasm and educational zeal to aspire to an idealized hospital with
a common ideology. This puts a strain on everyone and tends
to force people into being either for or against. [This factor
was difficult for me to assess, but I think to my supporters I
was acting as a facilitator, and to my detractors I was exerting
pressure (Jones, 1976a, pp. 27-38). This dilemma was in part
a factor in my growing awareness of the need for a truly objective facilitator and I think to some extent I succeeded in
achieving a more objective position. This transition in my
growth as a leader was greatly helped by the emergence of
multiple leadership as described later.] This polarization, I
think, is only a part truth because I feel I am liberal enough
to allow people to deviate, but there are and should be limits.
For example, Dr Small is tolerated to a remarkable degree and
no one expects her to conform, but her more outrageous sub-
terfuges *have* to be exposed if only to protect other people
from her influence, and to allow education to progress with
people who are open to learning. During the last two weeks
there have been signs that for the first time new-found
strength is being manifested in several staff members who can
enter into a difficult interpersonal wrangle - almost invariably
between two of the three senior people: Dr Morrice, Matron or
myself - and assume alternate leadership roles. This was the
unique characteristic of Henderson Hospital during the latter
part of my stay there, when three or four people could take
over when two of the senior staff members were locked in
angry discourse. I think my theory is reinforced by the fact
that, as I anticipated, the emergence of stronger doctors, in
the form of Dr Paul from the USA and Dr Shail Kumar from
India, has resulted in Dr Morrice feeling much more secure because they too are able to tackle me as equals. Dr Morrice

feels that his role as the leader of the opposition is often seen
as destructive when frequently this is not the case. There may
be considerable truth in this and it will be interesting to see
how things develop. [In retrospect I wonder how much of the
US sociologist's remarks had been heeded by me!]

During the last half of my second year at Dingleton I became
intimately involved with the geriatric wards. Dingleton was like
most psychiatric hospitals in that the centre of interest, training and change tended to be in the admission wards, whereas
the long-stay wards and particularly the geriatric wards tended
to receive relatively less attention. At this time we had on the
staff four trained psychiatrists, a senior house officer and a
part-time doctor locum. The latter was largely concerned with
the physical health of the old people, but was also very interested in psychiatry. Together we tried to look at the state of
the geriatric wards with a view to improving communication and,
as far as possible, helping patients and staff to come to some
decisions regarding their own organization and change. We
revitalized the usual ward meetings which were only appropriate
in the more articulate and less brain-damaged members of this
population. Almost 50 per cent of the patients in Dingleton were
65 years old or older, and most of them were classified as
geriatric.
   One of the factors which helped to revitalize the geriatric
wards was the presence of the activity assistants - young women
aged between 16 and $17\frac{1}{2}$ years, who organized the activity programme in the geriatric wards. This consisted of music and
movement, various simple games, community singing, reading to
the blind, and so on. We found that old people and teenagers
seemed to interact extremely well and the lack of self-consciousness
of the teenagers helped them to enter into music and movement
with an abandon which would have been difficult with older staff.
(Further discussion of the development of the activity assistant
programme is included in Chapter 3.)
   In August 1964 I noted in my 'Impressions':

On Friday the New Wing Group of old ladies showed some
distinct signs of becoming more alive. Mrs Gillespie talked
about wanting to find work outside. She had already been employed on our electronic work project in Galashiels and had
done well there. [As mentioned previously this was the only
project we attempted with an outside firm and was soon discontinued.] She now wants to find hotel or kitchen work in
the neighbourhood. The rehabilitation officer, Jim, was supposed to have done something about it, but we heard nothing
and he is now on leave. It was suggested she should do something herself, and look at advertisements in the local newspapers. The whole ward became interested, and various offers
were made to help her find work. This seems a very desirable
development to encourage initiative of this kind, when the

person has sufficient ego strength to undertake her own employment search.

The old ladies also raised the question of sedation, which we had talked about at a previous meeting. Apparently a number of them had not been turning up for their medication, and the charge nurse felt some concern and wanted to discuss the whole question of drugs. The nurse is making an up-to-date list of everyone's tranquillizers and other medications and Dr Black is planning to review this. However, it was suggested that it would be a very good thing if each patient were to indicate what she felt about her medication. The patients rejected the idea of this being done by the charge nurses asking each patient in turn, and preferred to hand in a note indicating their own preference. These notes are then to be considered in conjunction with the existing medication, and Dr Black will make whatever adjustments she thinks appropriate.

The patients discussed work in a more sensible way and felt that the important thing was not the pay, but the fact they were doing a useful job and felt they were earning their comfortable quarters and food. Some of them are working a full day and are getting relatively little pay. Others were getting more pay for less work, and it certainly would seem that we need to review the whole pay structure. What was so impressive was the growing activity among this group of old ladies and the fact that they have not given up the idea of moving out of the hospital to the outside community. At a previous discussion the patients had said that to have your medication withdrawn was dangerous, because it implied you were well enough to leave the hospital! This attitude seems to have changed for the better and a much more realistic atmosphere is apparent. I think if they had more admissions and discharges on this long-stay ward it would revitalize the whole climate.

By the end of October the geriatric wards were showing much more initiative.

On Thursday at our usual activity assistants meeting, they talked about some of their anxieties at work and about their fear of death and being faced by a dead person. After the meeting two of them came running back to say they had perhaps done something very naughty. Because of their curiosity they had asked one of the ward orderlies to let them see a dead person, or rather he had offered to show them one. They had done this and apparently felt relieved, but at the same time felt they might get this ward orderly into trouble and also felt guilty about what they had done. We reassured them this was a very enterprising and worthwhile attempt to relieve their anxieties about an unknown aspect of life. At the next meeting of the activity assistants we discussed their fear of death.

On Friday at the New Wing Geriatric meeting these same two

activity assistants were present, as was Annie Altschul, a
well-known British nursing instructor, who was visiting us.
It was a particularly interesting ward meeting in which we
discussed the way in which the patients have become less dependent on drugs, and most of them seemed to know exactly
why they got medicine and were anxious to use as little as
possible. I then asked them about the question of living outside, and mentioned the visits of the local authority and the
Medical Officer of Health from Peeblesshire the day before.
They were most emphatic about the need for people to live
outside the hospital in groups and were quite against the idea
of finding foster homes for individual patients. They said the
public would soon get tired of them and they would feel much
more secure if several of them were living together as a family
of old people. We discussed the possibility of getting them a
house in Melrose which they could run themselves. They were
most enthusiastic and ten of them volunteered for such a
project. Dr Black thought they would all be well enough to
take part in this project.

I then raised the question of Mrs Bruce who was absent
from the group. I was told she was very ill with pleurisy and
the patients had been visiting her in the infirmary ward. The
activity assistants had found Mrs Bruce to be a very difficult
patient before she became physically ill. She vetoed any
attempt on their part to get the other old ladies involved in
knitting groups, and in fact she seemed to negate everything.
Now we were told by Dr Black that she was very ill and she
seemed to have lost any desire to live. Dr Black wondered how
we could help to give Mrs Bruce more belief in her capacity to
recover. A discussion followed in which the old people showed
a great deal of wisdom and serenity. The activity assistants
were able to express their guilt at having been rather angry
with Mrs Bruce previously and now wished they could do something to repair any harm they may have caused her. Clearly
their anxiety linked up with the events of the activity assistants' meeting yesterday when they had been preoccupied with
death. Annie Altschul was amazed at the amount of communication that was occurring in a geriatric group and said that
she had never seen anything like it nor had she thought it
was possible.

The above illustrates how wise these old people can be about
their place in society. Their unwillingness to be placed in
families on their own and their insistence that they would fare
much better if they were allowed to live in groups anticipated
much of the current thinking about the placement of long-stay
patients. There was growing evidence that patients who had
lived together in hospital managed much better in the outside
community if they were allowed to continue their peer-group
relationship. It took us four years before we could act on this
early advice by the patients. We then helped them to become

established in two of our hospital houses and continue their com-
munal life, looking after their own needs.

Dingleton was paying more and more attention to the problem
of community psychiatry. In July 1964 a group of four staff went
to visit Dr Arthur Bowen who had established a splendid community psychiatric service in York. They had a weekly case conference involving the local authority and the hospital personnel.
Arthur Bowen himself had an appointment with the local authority,
as well as being the superintendent of the local mental hospital.
He told us that every patient was seen two weeks after leaving
hospital to make sure they were adjusting well to the community
at large. He was understandably proud of their pre-release unit
which was placed just outside the hospital and had fourteen
beds. Here female patients learned domestic skills and became
independent before they moved into the community itself. His
experience had convinced him that a mental health clinic was
best based on the local psychiatric hospital where the major resource personnel were found. His feeling was that until better
training was available for medical officers of health, family doctors and other people in the community, the mental health clinic
should not be run by the community outside. At the same time
he felt that in the long run community psychiatry would become
the province of social workers and others in the community.
Until more experience and better training was available, however,
the service was best integrated and run from the hospital itself.

It was during this period that I spent some time with Dr
Brotherston, the Chief Medical Officer for Scotland, formerly
Professor of Social Medicine at the Usher Institute in Edinburgh.
I found him a very forward-looking person who already saw the
possibilities of an integrated health service for the Borders. He
approved of our planning to develop health services in the
community and encouraged us to have a research worker to study
community attitudes. In fact, Joy Tuxford, who was visiting
Dingleton at that time, was encouraged to apply for this job
which materialized two years later.

A positive step forward in our community psychiatry practice
was the appointment of Iris Short to a post paid for by the local
authority, but based at Dingleton. This social worker was to do
an immensely valuable job in bridging the gap between Dingleton
and the local authority services in the community.

SUMMARY OF THE SECOND YEAR

The senior nursing staff, aided by the arrival of three new
colleagues who understood the aims of a therapeutic community,
began to take on leadership roles. They worked hard on a plan
to convert the two-shift (twelve-hour) system to a three-shift
(eight-hour) system. Working with this plan and involving as
many nurses as possible, but ineptly bypassing the night staff,
we learned much about our lack of skill in achieving consensus

on such a global issue. Despite many attempts over a three-month
period we achieved no tangible result. We asked the nurses to
present their own plan but when they did this, Matron ruled it
unworkable and was supported by the other senior nurses who
had raised the issue in the first place. Under pressure, the
junior nurses themselves seemed to be split with an unknown
number wanting no change. This issue was not resolved during
my seven years at Dingleton, although a three-shift system was
adopted later. Clearly, our ideal of achieving consensus proved
to be unworkable at this time with such a large group of over a
hundred nurses.

In general it might be said that consensus is an abstraction
useful only when a group of ten to twenty people, or less, with
considerable experience in problem-solving (group-work training
management theory, social learning, etc.) can conceptualize what
is entailed (Jones, 1968a, pp. 48-67; 1976a, pp. 57-9). No one
gets exactly what he or she wants and group goals take precedence over individual desires. Such sophistication was certainly
absent in the situation described, but probably applied to the
original plan conceptualized by a small group of senior nurses.

Many other factors were operating - mothers of young children
who liked a $4\frac{1}{2}$-day week, young men who could augment their
salaries with other work, etc. To identify these numerous variables would have been virtually impossible, and taken up an
absurd amount of time and with no useful outcome. We were
learning the hard way! Even so, nursing morale was rising
thanks to better recruitment, which was not unrelated to a much
better training programme.

It is interesting to note that at this period in our evolution to
an open system we openly retained the power of veto in order to
keep control over what we (the senior administration) might
regard as an unwise or irresponsible decision. When viewed
retrospectively we were still insecure enough to stop short of
full trust in the system. In other words we (the administration)
were not yet ready to relinquish some degree of control. Ultimately we became prepared to spend relatively large blocks of
time to achieve consensus on an important issue. These factors
may have contributed to our failure to reach consensus over the
issue of an eight-hour working day for nurses.

The first half of the second year saw daily community meetings
of all patients and staff established on all wards. These were
part of a move toward much greater patient responsibility,
especially in relation to their peers. Patients tend to ignore
patients to an extraordinary degree, so we were at least identifying patients as people with potential at this early stage. Staff
training still took priority, on the basic assumption that unless
the staff on a ward could interact effectively with their peers,
they had no right to be treating patients. But we were still a
long way from the kind of group training for all levels of staff
needed to realize such an ideal.

It was eighteen months after my arrival before serious problem

of leadership were identified and tackled (Jones, 1968a, pp. 23–47). I have dealt with my relationship with Dr Ken Morrice, my senior colleague, at considerable length in this chapter. This is done because it represents a familiar problem when only two people share most of the responsibility and authority, and both are psychiatrists. Ken, a competent and well-trained psychiatrist, was a great source of strength to his unit and indirectly to the hospital as a whole. He had been on the staff for seven years and gave continuity to the leadership. The more established 'old guard' knew where they were with him and so the appeal of the familiar was strong and contrasted inevitably with my new approach. At the same time Ken was identified with and welcomed a therapeutic community approach. However, the ubiquitous Dr Small, a member of his team but still identified with the entire hospital through night duties which she chose and which we gratefully allowed her to monopolize, was a rallying point for the forces of reaction. With no formal training in psychiatry she tried to please everyone, at the same time controlling deviant behaviour with a moralistic fervour. Naturally many of the nursing staff liked her method of avoiding trouble. There is no way of knowing to what extent her devious ways helped to drive a wedge between Ken and myself, but her loyalty to him did not help me!

Almost inevitably Ken was cast in the mould of the leader of the opposition, an essential factor in any democracy, and a role that he played superbly. Honest, outspoken and afraid of no one, he helped to uncover endless covert problems, a process which helped enormously in our growth. Unfortunately, as with parental problems, it was difficult to remain objective when one was emotionally involved. A third party acceptable to the two main characters was needed as a facilitator. Lacking this at the time in question, we must have missed many valuable opportunities for social learning. All too often we merely debated, or if emotions were high, quarrelled, and so little or no learning occurred (Jones, 1976a, pp. 43–53).

During this second year we tended to focus on staff training on the job' rather than in more formal lectures. This upset some of the young student nurses whose first priority was to pass exams, which meant higher status and pay. However, living situations were gaining momentum and had an enormous effect on ward morale and interdisciplinary understanding. Learning as a social process took precedence over teaching in a lecture room. However, teaching and learning as a social process were seen as complementary.

The rapid change in the culture at Dingleton made severe demands on some of the more entrenched staff, and in particular the Matron who felt she was in danger of being ridiculed by the matrons of other hospitals whose power over their nursing staffs remained supreme. She was nearing retirement and pictured herself as a leper in her own profession. In fact this never happened, but situations such as these, the inevitable by-products

of change, were not uncommon and aroused anxiety in everyone
and we coined the clause 'learning is a painful process!'

A staff nurse, Reg, was invaluable as an example of a 'risk-
taker' throughout my whole time at Dingleton. This concept is
an essential part of an open system and is a complementary part
of confrontation (Jones, 1976a, pp. 42-3, 122). Reg realized
during the first few weeks of my stay that I cherished risk-
takers who, by their challenge of authority, tested out the
administrator's good faith in not taking reprisals when negative
feelings toward authority were openly expressed. All too often
people in authority invite free expression of feelings: 'Say anything you like', only to use this 'honesty' against the risk-taker
at some future date. A risk-taker can communicate feelings befor
a high level of trust makes this 'safe' for others to do so, thus
contributing significantly to the rate of change. I felt the need
to protect Reg from reprisal on occasion and it is to Matron's
credit that she understood this aspect of my role as time went on
and was herself able ultimately to curb her temptation to 'put
down' a critic. In fact positive criticism is an essential ingredien
of learning as a social process. The word criticism has come to
have a negative connotation and we do not have a word that
conveys the idea of positive criticism. The transactional analysts
use of the word 'strokes' has a limited meaning, and does not
adequately convey the idea of a thoughtful appraisal of the content, but rather an emotional response. In fact we seem to find
it much easier to find fault than to recognize the positive meanin
in situations - as the right/wrong dichotomy of our schooldays,
where emphasis on 'success' influences our thinking and judgment to seek out the negative when asked to give an evaluation.
In the classroom, commenting on a peer's behaviour is seen as
telling 'tattle tales'. Even positive criticism in the context of
social learning often conveys more pain than pleasure. It takes a
brave person to comment without reservation about another person's performance. But to learn how one's behaviour appears to
an interested observer is to learn about one's own subjective
distortions and ego defences. In this sense painful communicatio
is an essential part of social learning. The 'risk-taker' role
applies to such an individual who, like Reg, came to realize that
everyone needs to know the difference between how he subjec-
tively perceives himself and how he appears to an objective
observer. (Obviously no one is totally 'objective'; objectivity is
relative, as is 'open' in reference to open and closed systems.)
Had the environment not been a trusting one, Reg would have
been 'muzzled' and his potential unused.

The problems of leadership already alluded to at the early par
of the second year began to improve as that year ended. Two
other experienced psychiatrists, one from the US and the other
from India, joined the staff. This meant that if Ken Morrice and
I were in conflict as so often happened, one or both of the new
psychiatrists was in a relatively uninvolved or objective position
and could play the role of facilitator. This was an immense relie

:o Ken and myself, not to mention the other staff members present. These alternate leaders also acted as role models for other
>otential leaders, for example, some senior members of the
1ursing staff. So a pattern emerged which amounted to a
`acilitator being available at all times when emotional issues sur-
aced at the SSC or when a crisis erupted in any part of the
1ospital (Jones, 1976a, pp. 27-38). Dr Paul Polak was to stay
with us for two years and we refined our concepts of crisis
ntervention during this time (Jones and Polak, 1968).

The increase in the number of experienced psychiatrists also
neant that I was free to move from the admission wards to the
ess popular geriatric wards. With the help of a female doctor,
he nurses and the young activity assistants we were able to
lemonstrate the value of therapeutic community principles to this
irea. Thus, the patients on a female ward asked if each of them
:ould hand in a note to the charge nurse indicating their prefer-
:nce for or against a sedative, and these preferences would be
·onsidered as the doctor reviewed their existing medication, mak-
ng whatever final adjustments she thought fit. At one ward
1eeting the old ladies amazed us by their firm conviction that
hey should return to the outside community when possible. But
hey were against the idea of foster homes for individual patients,
 long-standing tradition in Scotland, and thought they would
are much better in a disinterested world if several of them chose
o live together as a family of old people. This, in fact, material-
zed four years later and was the patients' own version of Fair-
reather's famous lodges (Fairweather et al., 1974).

As the therapeutic community in the hospital took shape, we
·egan to turn our attention to the development of similar prin-
iples in the outside community of the Borders. Our involvement
·ith the 68 family doctors who served the Borders community
rew, as did our liaison with the public health and local author-
:ies.

Chapter 3

The third year, 1965:
confrontation in high places

INTRODUCTION

A therapeutic community represents a relatively integrated
social organization. Ideally, the regional central authority no
longer controls the hospital administrative system, where previously efficiency meant the immediate and expeditious response
to instructions from above. The concept of a therapeutic community implies the involvement of all personnel in the aims and
practices of the organization. The hospital is no longer an
'obedient child', but questions and is at all times potentially
rebellious.

We started our third year well aware of the fact that our evolutionary progress toward an open system might strain our
relationship with the central authority at two levels (Jones,
1976a, pp. 3-15): (a) our own Hospital Board of Management
made up of local dignitaries from the small town of Melrose and
the surrounding area; and (b) the South-Eastern Regional
Health Board located in Edinburgh, which controlled all the
hospitals in the south-eastern part of Scotland. Little did we
realize that this year would also involve enquiry and interaction
with the highest authority in Scotland in the form of the Secreta
of State and the Health Authority for Scotland situated in St
Andrew's House in Edinburgh.

CONFRONTATION IN HIGH PLACES

Our relationship with the Board of Management had been remark
ably harmonious up to this time, but some ruffling of the smoott
waters was inevitable. The only incident of this kind that I recorded in the first two years concerned the 'open day and fair'
including a band of Highland pipers and a sheep-herding demon
stration held on the last Saturday of August 1964. We had abou
1,500 visitors and made a profit of almost £500 on the stalls,
raffle, and so on. The main emphasis was on helping the community learn about the hospital and the majority of people did a
complete tour of the wards, talking with patient and staff guide
Everyone appeared to have a thoroughly good time and the tea-
room staffed by patients was a great success. The atmosphere
was one of gaiety - very different to the visitors' expectations.
The day was essentially a hospital affair and the Board of Mana
ment felt somewhat overshadowed because they were not involve

in the planning. At the next board meeting the chairman of the
Board of Management felt the Regional Board should be told of
the profit we had made, and wondered if we were justified in
using this money for hospital amenities! At a deeper level I felt
that because things seemed to be changing fairly rapidly and
arousing a considerable amount of interest in the world at large,
the Board of Management felt somewhat bypassed. The fact is
they had been most supportive, sanctioning all kinds of change,
but feeling themselves to be in the role of spectators rather
than initiators. The most critical of the board members was one
who had most contact with the patients and knew the hospital
practices in some detail. He had a good relationship with several
of the nurses socially and tended to feed back grievances to the
board meetings without discussing these grievances with myself
or the Matron.

A frank discussion of our difficulties seemed worth trying and
I met this board member, along with one of my senior colleagues,
in the hope of achieving a learning situation. The board member
accepted our invitation, but made it clear from the start that he
was ultra-conservative, and disapproved of our rapid liberal-
ization of the hospital structure. He disagreed with me that he
was playing a dual role of championing the nurses and at the
same time trying to be an objective board member. However, he
did agree that the area of patient treatment was entirely the
province of the staff. I tried to show him that he was in danger
of picking up rumours and statements of an ill-digested kind and
of feeding these back to the board meetings without the kind of
analysis which the staff did daily through the Senior Staff
Committee or ward meetings. I cited a current rumour implying
that I approved of sexual relations among the patients, which
was patently ludicrous, but nevertheless was apparently believed
by some of the staff. I think we were able to establish very
definite lines of demarcation between our respective roles, and
by implication between the role of a board member and a member
of the clinical staff. I was certain this discussion led to a better
understanding between us, and he no longer behaved in the
board meetings as though he was a special representative of the
nursing or patient population. Instead, he played a valuable
opposition role, questioning proposed changes in a way which
allowed the board to understand better what we were trying to
do.

Another example of using the technique of confrontation with
those in authority occurred regarding our activity assistant
scheme, which we created during the second year. I am including this information in this chapter because it forms the background to the events of confrontation with the Regional Board
which occurred in our third year.

Up to this point I had had no significant contact with the
Regional Board situated in Edinburgh, 35 miles from Melrose,
who were not only our employers, but who were responsible to
the Secretary of State for Scotland for the effective running of

Dingleton Hospital. At the beginning of my second year the
chairman of the Regional Board had been kind enough to invite
me to an informal dinner, where we had talked about Dingleton
and its future in a very friendly way. In the second year we
began to think about a new plan for improving nurse recruitment. We tried all the familiar approaches such as writing
articles in the nursing and medical press (Jones and Dewer,
1964; Jones, 1964; 1963), advertising extensively, and tried to
get away from the usual stereotyped nurse advertisement to
something more exciting. In addition, we sent our nurse tutor to
various centres of employment in Ireland, and had responded to
every approach from outside organizations for talks, discussions
etc. We did our utmost to encourage schools in our neighbourhood to visit us and we were prepared to visit them.

We noticed that the early school-leavers, aged 15 or 16 years
old, usually tended to drift into employment in the local tweed
mills which offered immediate prospects of a reasonable salary,
but poor long-term prospects for advancement. The minimum age
for nurse recruitment in Scotland was $17\frac{1}{2}$, but by this time most
of the early school-leavers were already established in jobs. We
felt to bridge this gap might solve our recruitment difficulties
and also afford young people an interesting experience of hospital work. It also allowed them to delay their final choice of
career until they were more certain about what they wanted.

We raised this whole matter in January 1964 and with the
approval of our Board of Management began to advertise posts
which we designated 'Activity Assistant'. Our first application
was received in April 1964, and by June the scheme was properly
under way. The scheme was limited to eight young women and
was deliberately planned so they were not involved in 'nursing'
duties. Their role was to help interest and activate the geriatric
patients, and, when requested, to help the nurses with bed-
making, etc., but always under their supervision. They were
also given opportunities to experience other hospital activities
such as the kitchen, laundry, clerical work, canteen, etc. A
young college student attached to the social work department
acted as their mentor and confidante, and they were also under
the jurisdiction of the nurse tutor.

At the end of October 1964 we had a visit from some of the
senior officials from the Regional Board in Edinburgh who wanted
to discuss the activity assistant programme with representatives
of our own Board of Management. They claimed we had launched
this programme without consulting them. This was true, but they
were informed of our decision as they automatically received
minutes of our own hospital board meetings where the programme
had been discussed and sanctioned. We were told we were in
danger of exploiting young people and this was against the policy
of Scottish nursing. In England there was a Cadet Nurse scheme
but this was not acceptable to the Scottish nursing bodies. I
suggested the visitors might like to meet the activity assistants
themselves, as these young women would give them a much better

account of their activities and feelings than we could. The offer
was ignored. We also pointed out that we felt this was an important breakthrough in psychiatric nurse recruitment and could
well benefit all psychiatric hospitals in the country.

The visitors seemed far from pleased, said we could not yet
call the programme an official one, and in fact denied us the
right to recruit further until we had permission from the Regional
Board. The Matron, although not directly responsible for the
programme, spoke very positively in its favour. The girls could
not be under her jurisdiction because we knew that Scottish
nursing bodies were against the employment of young people
in mental hospitals, so we were careful not to make this a nursing programme.

In December, having had no word from the Regional Board as
yet, we held a meeting with the activity assistants and their
relatives. The latter were extremely enthusiastic about the programme, and had no criticism whatsoever to offer. Sharing with
them the opposition we were receiving from the nursing structure
in Scotland, they said they would do all they could to help us
as they regarded the programme an important development in
education.

The above incidents are recorded because they form a prelude
to a series of events which, although very painful, were probably
a necessary evolutionary step in our own relationship as a hospital with the Regional Board. I would like to think they demonstrate the possibility of using techniques of confrontation and
social learning in relation to external problems as well as those
limited to the hospital.

During the week ending 13 February 1965, the Board of
Management was requested to send a deputation to meet certain
officials of the Regional Board regarding the activity assistant
programme and 'certain other matters'. We had heard on the
grapevine that rumours about our moral standards at Dingleton
were circulating in Edinburgh. Jimmy Millar and three members
of our Board of Management and myself listened to the chairman
of this ad-hoc committee of the Regional Board who told us about
unconfirmed rumours which were of a sufficiently serious nature
to force the Regional Board to do something. Apparently similar
rumours had reached the Home and Health Department, the highest medical authority in Scotland. We were told these rumours
had been discussed at a meeting of the Regional Nurse Training
Committee and that a prominent matron of a teaching hospital
had said that she was not prepared to second any of her nurses
for psychiatric training at Dingleton. Rumour had it that several
of our nurses had become pregnant and that patients were involved. The chairman of the Regional Nurse Training Committee
was told by the Secretary of State for Scotland that he could not
accept our activity assistant scheme in its present form and that
the programme was suspended. Knowing of our nurse shortage,
it was stated that if necessary, wards would have to be closed in
order to maintain at least a minimum service! The chairman spoke

for about twenty minutes and we were simply appalled. It seemed to us that the situation was prejudiced without even hearing our point of view. The rumours were treated as fact, and already an action was taken to suspend the activity assistant scheme. The chairman admitted that he had no evidence that any of the rumours had emanated from the Borders, and that all the talk had come from Edinburgh which was 35 miles away. In fact he had himself sounded out one or two people in the Borders and received no indication of trouble from this enquiry.

The chairman of our Board of Management responded that these were very serious allegations, all based on rumour, and that it was difficult for us to reply without knowing the people who were perpetrating these tales. We were told that these names were not to be divulged! I expressed concern and anger at the way the situation was handled. We told the Regional Board that we knew of only two pregnancies with student nurses over the past ten years. I wondered if this might be better than the record of any other hospital in Scotland! It seemed a pity that this was somehow linked with the activity assistant programme, implying that these women were being exposed to immoral influence. I expressed my feelings that this approach to recruitment was of such importance from the national point of view that I intended to take the matter to the Secretary of State for Scotland acting as a private citizen and not as the Physician Superintendent of Dingleton. We had just begun to find a way to redress our serious shortage of nurses and instead of appreciation we received a rebuff. It seemed to me a great pity that the people judging this issue had never even met the activity assistants, although there had been several occasions when this might have been done without any inconvenience. For the nursing hierarchy to have had such strong opinions about 16-year-old girls being 'exposed to circumstances prevailing in a mental hospital' seemed unrealistic. In my opinion they were probably subjected to greater stresses in the tweed mills and similar occupations which were their other work alternatives. The chairman repeatedly talked about their nursing duties, and we pointed out this as inaccurate because the scheme explicitly avoided 'nursing'; they were merely helping with feeding old people, accompanying patients for walks, bed-making, and so on.

It is difficult to say if this angry exchange between the team from the hospital meeting their employers achieved very much as a learning situation (Jones, 1968a, pp. 68-74). It was, however, an important occasion because we had made our position perfectly clear, and expressed surprise and anger that the Regional Board and the Home and Health Department had paid so much attention to rumour, initiating action before hearing and understanding our point of view. It was fairly reasonable to suppose that at least some members of the Regional Board were piqued because we showed initiative and acted on our own behalf without approval from them. Had we asked their approval it seemed highly probable that the whole matter would have been shelved; at least the

resistance and negative reaction of the meeting indicated this
was a strong possibility. At the meeting I made the point that
our free communication network and willingness to expose our
problems for open discussion and learning made the staff at
Dingleton very vulnerable. This applied particularly to visitors
who were professional people and were assumed to have respect
for the group's confidentiality and trust that was extended to
them.

   In retrospect I think we learned the danger of such a system
of open communication with visitors or trainees when there was
little opportunity to work through and process situations, etc.
We took it for granted that new staff members would be uncomfortable with our techniques of crisis intervention, confrontation
and living-learning situations. These involved everyone present
at meetings and required considerable training in group dynamics and therapeutic community principles before one could achieve
the degree of understanding and objectivity which were an
integral part of the learning process. We had reason to believe
this particular rumour (about pregnancies) was sparked off by
three fairly senior general trained nurses who had spent three
weeks at Dingleton as part of a training course. They were
very upset by the open discussion of day-to-day problems and
the absence of the familiar disciplinary machinery which protected most people in the social system from involvement. The
immediate response of these three visitors, who were accustomed
to the authority system of a general hospital, was to talk about
their experience at Dingleton and seek reassurance and support
from their seniors when they returned to their training course
in Edinburgh. To the hospital system generally, Dingleton
stood for change, and was a threat to the whole nursing authority system in Scotland. The clash of cultures between a
general hospital and the open system at Dingleton often presented difficulties and led to misunderstanding. Nurses in
general hospitals are protected by the nursing hierarchy and
difficult situations are automatically referred to the appropriate
level of line authority.

   Although painful for us, this experience was probably an
important aspect of any process of change that might occur in
a hospital system in Scotland. It seemed important to us to
demonstrate that we must not passively accept the Regional
Board's criticism. To turn this experience of prejudice into a
learning situation we had to be active, and use confrontation
with all the skill we could muster. This process had, in a sense,
been started when I made it clear that I intended to see the
Secretary of State for Scotland, or some high official, as a
citizen rather than as the Physician Superintendent. I made it
quite explicit that I wanted to discuss our plans for nurse
recruitment, and how I felt these were being blocked in a negative way by the Regional Board.

   I also took it upon myself to interact with our most angry
critic, a Regional Board member, after the meeting. He hinted

darkly of the danger that the whole matter would get to the
press, and implied that this was why we had a hearing with an
ad-hoc committee rather than one of the formal committees to
which the press were admitted. I questioned his assumption
that press intervention would be catastrophic, because if the
inquiry was carried out with any thoroughness, Dingleton would
have everything to gain. My aim was to attempt to achieve some
degree of understanding of this man's point of view, and if
possible engage his interest in this approach to nurse recruitment. I think I partly succeeded in dispelling his own fantasies
about the exploitation of the young, and in dealing with the
problem facing recruitment for psychiatric hospitals in general.
This technique of personal confrontation after the 'formal' meeting caught our severest critic 'off guard'. He was forced not
only to look at his own preconceptions, but he was not allowed
to hide behind his role as an ad-hoc committee member of a
powerful political group, but had to deal on a 'man-to-man'
personal level with me where he knew his armour was useless.

The next week brought to light several factors which partially
justified the action of the Regional Board and aroused some
awareness of the inadequacies of our own communication system.
The Matron, without consulting her two senior colleagues, Mr
Millar and myself, took the chairman of our Board of Management
to see the male nurses' home. The student nurses were supposed to make their beds, but the place was in a state of chaos
and there were numerous beer bottles scattered around in a
way which invited fantasy. Embarrassed, the Matron apparently
described her difficult situation in relation to discipline and
morality at Dingleton. Understandably enough, she blamed me
as the initiator of the therapeutic community, and said I made
light of situations concerning morality.

The chairman's anxiety was sufficiently high for him to call a
meeting of the Dingleton Hospital Board members who had participated in the confrontation with the Regional Board, myself
and Dr Morrice. The Dingleton Board chairman started by talking about rumours and said that it was clear we were not going
to get anywhere until we were in possession of the facts which
the Regional Board had refused to divulge. We discussed the
situation in the male nurses' home which had been witnessed
by the chairman and the Matron. She cited an instance when
two staff members were seen leaving the nurses' home at 5.00
a.m., and implied that I had completely ignored this. In actual
fact, my recollection was quite the opposite and I was surprised
and rather impressed by the fact that the Matron had not made
a major issue of this incident at its occurrence, and which I
only heard about later. Even so, such behaviour should have
been fed back to the SSC, and the two people concerned should
have been participants in a living-learning situation. We could
not condone such behaviour but might have turned it into a
learning situation in order to avoid other incidents of this kind.
It was clear that the Matron was not comfortable with such learn

ing situations, and felt, quite understandably, that the therapeutic community disapproved of her using her traditional disciplinary role as the head of the nursing system.

My colleague, Ken Morrice, having been at Dingleton much
longer than I, expressed the opinion that the moral tone of the
hospital was much better now than at any time during the eight
years he had been on the staff. He felt that, following my
arrival, there had been a state of transition when people had
been confused and mistook permissive ideas for licence. I added
that I recalled a time when the patients thought that allowing
the sexes to mix would result in a lot of pregnancies, and they
had talked about giving some of the offspring my name! The
chairman felt the two pregnant nurses who were the main source
of the rumours could not possibly be attributed to me because
they antedated the system which I had initiated.

The discussion turned to the tendency to link pregnancies
among nurses with the activity assistant scheme. It was felt that
the nursing profession in general seemed to resist the idea of
young people in hospitals; but anticipating this difficulty we
explicitly kept the activity assistants outside the formal control
of the nursing profession. The activity assistants were in a
position to question much of what they saw in the hospital without fear of reprisal. They had frequent, and latterly daily,
seminars with staff members from various disciplines, and represented a challenge to any 'closed' system which might develop
on a particular ward.

During the discussion I pointed out that I felt fairly certain
that behind all the rumours was a personal attack on myself, but
more particularly on my ideas. I had encountered similar resistance, first at Henderson Hospital in London and later in Oregon
Hospital in the USA, because the democratic egalitarian social
structure of a therapeutic community threatened the authority
of an established hierarchical hospital system.

This discussion was a valuable learning situation and improved
relations and understanding among the senior officials in both
the Board of Management and in the hospital. We agreed on the
need for the nurses to take more responsibility for their own
behaviour and discipline, and that we, the hospital, should
report back to the Regional Board giving full details of our
findings. I was also encouraged to continue my plans to see the
Under-Secretary of State for Scotland, with a view to recon-
stituting the activity assistant scheme.

We learned the name of the matron at an Edinburgh hospital
who had expressed disapproval of the morals at Dingleton and
would not allow her nurses to be seconded here. In pursuance
of our policy to try and turn rumour into a learning situation,
the Matron and I went to see this woman. She turned out to be
most courteous, and gave us an excellent lunch with some particularly good sherry! She said that she felt she was acting res-
ponsibly by raising the rumours about Dingleton at the Regional
Board Nursing Committee meeting. We replied that the Regional

Board had acted on these rumours as though they had foundation in fact, instead of making adequate enquiries. The discussion was carried out in a fairly friendly way and certainly helped a great deal to clear up misunderstanding.

At the SSC the following day we agreed to pursue seeking face-to-face confrontation with some of the senior officers of the Regional Board. This was easily arranged as we were required to feed back our findings in relation to the rumours and supposed misdemeanours at Dingleton. At this meeting I expressed our conviction that the rumours were ridiculous; that the two pregnancies had occurred prior to my arrival and had no relevance to the present scene. I repeated that the rumours in Edinburgh seemed to have no counterpart in the Borders, and asked that the question of nursing morals be kept quite apart from the problem of the activity assistant scheme. Our Matron talked with feeling about the indignities to which she was being subjected. When she met other senior nurses in Edinburgh they asked her what she was doing about the babies, referring apparently to the supposed progeny of patients at Dingleton! She hinted at the possibility of seeking legal advice. We implied that we were the injured party and not the Regional Board. We were told the slate would be wiped clean, as we had convinced everyone there was little foundation for the rumours about Dingleton. However, we also were informed that there was little chance of the activity assistant scheme being accepted in its present form. We pointed out the inconsistency of these statements, and that if they were now satisfied then surely they would recommend to the Home and Health Department the re-establishment of the activity assistant scheme. The representative of the Home and Health Department who was present tried to act as peace-maker, suggested that time was a great healer, and if the matter was allowed to rest everything would come out alright! I mentioned that I had received an acknowledgment to my letter from the Under-Secretary of State for Scotland, and ended with another recommendation that our critics meet the activity assistants and familiarize themselves with the situation at first hand.

The following day I met two of the senior doctors at the Home and Health Department and had a very fair hearing. They felt it would be wiser to see the activity assistant scheme in the context of nursing recruitment, and have one of the senior nursing staff as a supervisor of the programme. I enquired about our suggestion that the Regional Board should be invited to come and see the activity assistants for themselves, but they felt it was far better to let the whole matter cool off. They added that the chairman of the Regional Board was very positive about Dingleton and liked our experimental attitude.

The crisis surrounding the activity scheme, the supposed immorality of our nurses and our response in the form of various discussions and confrontation all occurred within a period of three weeks. In actual fact, a member of the Home and Health Department visited three weeks later and had a long interview with the

activity assistants on his own. They reported he had been quite
charming and very understanding. Two months later, toward the
end of May 1965, we heard unofficially from the Regional Board
that the activity assistant scheme would probably be re-
established, but with a senior nurse in charge.

On 5 July 1965 we had a visit from some of the senior members
of the South-Eastern Scotland Regional Hospital Board who met
some of our own Board of Management and senior staff. Incidental
to this meeting, the chairman and secretary of the Regional
Board had an informal discussion with the five activity assistants
remaining in post and learned that they had all decided to take
up psychiatric nursing. The Regional Board members expressed
themselves as greatly impressed with these young women. We explained that at present they were jointly supervised by a nurse
tutor, a deputy matron and a social worker. We were asked to
guarantee the welfare of the activity assistants from a moral
point of view and their non-employment in male geriatric wards,
even in an emergency! They added, however, that formal permission still awaited discussions between the Regional Board and
the Home and Health Department.

On 13 July we had a letter from the Regional Board indicating
their agreement to recommend the Scottish Home and Health
Department the continuation of the activity assistant scheme as
an experiment. This experiment was to be carried out by recruit-
ing up to ten activity assistants, not under 16 years of age, who
would work in various departments of the hospital, such as
occupational therapy, music and movement, the laundry and kitchen, and in female geriatric wards and female long-stay wards.
Our instructions were: their duties should not include work in
male wards of any kind; they should not take part in group
therapy discussion anywhere in the hospital; Matron should be
designated as directly responsible to the Board of Management
for the general welfare of the activity assistants; and immediate
consideration should be given to the inclusion of some form of
further education in the work/experiential programme. Finally,
there would be a review of the whole scheme in July 1966.

Final approval of the scheme reached us in August 1965, nine
months after the initial intervention from higher authorities. It
was a long, arduous, time-consuming exercise which taught us
something about the ways of bureaucracy, and we hoped had
been a valuable learning experience for some people in authority
as well.

LIVING-LEARNING SITUATIONS FOR STAFF

Living-learning situations may occur quite spontaneously in
ordinary ward life when a crisis occurs and the problem is discussed immediately by the people concerned (Jones, 1968a, pp.
87-90). More often, however, some skilled group worker from
another area of the hospital is invoked in order to create some

degree of objectivity, and to give the situation a structure in which optimal learning may occur. In regularly scheduled staff seminars, sensitivity training groups, or reviews after ward groups, very similar learning situations present themselves. (Sensitivity training groups were an important aspect of staff training. A homogeneous group of eight or ten staff, for example student nurses, with an experienced group worker acting as a facilitator met weekly for one hour and learned how to express feelings of frustration, rivalry, etc., in the presence of their peers, and thus learned at first hand about process and social learning.) In the previous section on confrontation in high places the value of using situations for learning opportunities, even at a high administrative level, was indicated. Under such circumstances there is inevitably a much greater time-lag than is desirable within the circumscribed area of the hospital. Timing is very important. Although painful, a confrontation should be arranged immediately following a crisis, when feelings, interest and motivation to resolve the difficulty are still high. A delay even of hours may mean that many rationalizations and other defences are mobilized.

An example of social learning through confrontation, precipitated by a group of visitors who came for a day, is as follows:

On Monday we had a visit from Dr Edwards from a nearby psychiatric hospital and his psychology department with about eight students. They spent the morning in treatment groups and at two o'clock we had a seminar with the visitors and some of our own staff. This was a tense, uncomfortable meeting, where we had difficulty in finding common ground. The psychologists were a bit abstract, and talked about statistics and results, as well as learning theory. There was little evidence that they had much understanding of what we were trying to accomplish. At three o'clock I left to go to my weekly training meeting with the student nurses. One of the psychologists and several of the students chose to come with me. When we got to the seminar the student nurses were asked if we could join them, and they said 'no'. We were forced to withdraw, and then talked quite comfortably for about twenty minutes, because we had all been rejected and this somehow brought us closer together. I then suggested we might try to create a face-to-face confrontation.

I returned to the seminar room and asked the student nurses if we could join them now. They agreed, and indicated that they had spent twenty minutes letting off steam. They said they were extremely angry with me because I had been away a great deal recently in America and Europe, and they felt rejected. Moreover, I had arrived seven minutes late for their seminar and had brought a lot of strangers with me. They were fed up with visitors who seemed to take up all my time, and they were beginning to feel the regular nurses were not very important. They then talked about the transient nurses [visitors]

who might be here for a few days or months, and who were
given many of the interesting learning situations. I explained
this was a very difficult issue and I entirely sympathized with
them. When someone was sent from, say, Finland, to learn
therapeutic community methods, it was difficult not to put
them in a ward where they could have an optimal learning
experience. I was accused of being much more interested in
the transients than in the regular staff. They described many
cliques in the hospital, and then switched to a discussion of
the meagre opportunity for social life afforded by a rural
hospital. In discussing what we could do about this problem it
soon became clear that we [the hospital] could not be held
responsible for their private lives, but we did agree that
sharing the interest of the work should be carefully considered
They admitted that in the past some of the work therapists had
been very generous about relieving them to go to seminars
and teaching sessions, but this co-operation had somehow
fallen into disuse. We agreed to have a face-to-face confrontation the following week, and invite all seven work therapists
to attend. In this way it is hoped we can bring about some
kind of equilibration between the work therapists who can fit
in most meetings in their programme and the student nurses
who are tied to a more rigid schedule.

After the meeting I discussed the possibility of having a
social evening once a month which the Matron and Kerstin, my
wife, might be responsible for, and which could be held at
our home on the hospital grounds. This was agreed to and we
have put in the newsletter an invitation for next Thursday at
8.00 p.m. It will be interesting to see how far this social
occasion is used by the more lonely nursing personnel. We also
hope some of the married nurses will use this opportunity to
get closer to the senior staff. I think the whole question of
social relationships is a two-way process, and neither the
senior staff nor the regular nurses are wholly responsible.
They probably want a good deal of independence in their
private lives, but at least the opportunity for interaction
should be made available.

I think this seminar with the student nurses, and the way in
which it was turned into a living-learning situation, is a good
example of what we mean by the term 'confrontation'. The
effect on the psychology visitors was quite dramatic. They
immediately enthused about Dingleton and what we were trying
to do, and said this actual demonstration had helped them to
understand our theoretical framework. [It might also be said
that by returning a second time with the visitors to the
students' seminar, I was abusing my authority! Or was I
acting as a risk-taker?]

LIVING-LEARNING SITUATIONS FOR PATIENTS

I would like to describe the stage we had reached in developing living-learning situations by the end of 1965 with an illustration which involves the patients.

On Tuesday we had a very interesting ward meeting in Female Ward IV. This long-stay ward is beginning to verbalize the things that go on in the patients' own private world. We were talking about two patients (a man and a woman) falling in love with each other, and in the review afterwards one of the post-graduate nurses was able to say she had seen two patients on the men's side who were masturbating each other. She had not known what to do with this information, had simply told the charge nurse and left it at that. We are seeing how difficult it is even for nurses to talk about things which go on outside their familiar culture, but I think we are moving a step closer to understanding the sexual culture that exists in the long-stay population. It was quite clear the nurses were not sufficiently comfortable to allow such information to come out with any degree of freedom. I left the meeting thinking about the inevitable sexual frustration long-stay patients must feel and wondered if we should perhaps legitimize some forms of sexual outlet.

This impression regarding sexual prejudice was reinforced at the Thursday combined ward meeting of Lounge One and Female Ward IV, where about sixty male and female patients meet together. This meeting was remarkable in the extent to which the patients hinted at private behaviour. They managed to talk about Alfred, a scraggy little epileptic, who apparently washes himself every morning in the nude. Some patients described this as disgusting, but apparently they had become used to it. The nurses recalled that years ago Alfred had indulged in some kind of homosexual activities with a mongoloid. It was also reported that some female patients in Ward IV walk about naked in the washroom, and again this was described as disgusting. It was even hinted at that some people slept in the nude! Patients seemed to be indicating that any deviation from a strict moral code might bring about dire consequences from the nursing staff. The patients also mentioned that staff had been invading the 'smoking corridor'. This is a remote area which male patients use to escape the formal life of the hospital, a dingy, dungeon-like basement. In the further recesses of this basement it is rumoured that homosexual activities have been known to occur. We had asked Anthea Boyd, a temporary social worker, to try to analyse the culture in the smoking passage, and she had given us an interesting paper. Nevertheless, her intrusion into this area had seemed to show that the staff were taking some kind of interest which was assumed to be disapproving in a private area of the male patients' lives.

In fact the SSC were intrigued by this private world which
schizophrenics used as a sanctuary and allowed them free rein
for their fantasies without being observed. It helped to give
them a group identity and we decided to respect their private
space. To study their behaviour in isolation would have been
impossible without destroying a place which they had created
as their own. Anthea Boyd's paper helped to reaffirm our feelings about allowing this place to remain as the patients wished.

> There is also the fact that we are talking about a complete re-
> organization of the hospital to bring about a much closer
> integration of male and female patients as well as male and
> female staff. Inevitably this must disturb patients a great
> deal, and although they did not say this quite explicitly, it
> is well known that they are talking a great deal about it, and
> show concern about increased proximity of the sexes. After
> many decades of segregation comes the more recent loosening
> of this isolation of the sexes.
>   It will be a long time before the patients fully realize that
> the staff would like them to develop their own culture in the
> wards and in the hospital generally.

So with patients it seemed that confrontation and learning as a
social process was as yet at an early stage of development compared with the staff. At this stage of our development we were
not including the patients in decision-making, even when it concerned them intimately.

INTRAMURAL DEVELOPMENTS

During January 1965 we established a weekly case conference
for teaching purposes, and every week rather than every month
the Journal Club met. Both these functions continued throughout
my stay, except that the focus of the Journal Club turned almost
entirely to topics of current interest or hearing of developments
in other places from visitors. In February the old canteen was
replaced by a new patient/staff canteen. This afforded a large
and very comfortable coffee shop where interaction of an informal
kind was greatly enhanced, and where patients could take their
visitors for a comfortable setting in which to chat. The service
was done entirely by the patients themselves and the profits
returned to patient amenities of one kind or another.

In November, after many hours of discussion with staff and
patients at all levels we initiated a new physical organization of
the hospital. This involved a redistribution of patients throughout the major part of the hospital to bring about a closer integration of the sexes with greater freedom for social interaction
than previously. I was in Europe at the time of the actual
physical reorganization, but was told the whole move took place
within two days. The patients were the deciding factor in pre-

cipitating the change. Inevitably there was a large and powerful
reactionary group led by one of the doctors who prophesied all
kinds of serious consequences which would result from the
mixing of the sexes. On my return I found that integration had
resulted in a remarkable effect on the hospital. Patients were
interacting much more freely than they had done in the past.
Annabel, a patient who had been one of the loudest to protest
about the move from the nice old ladies' ward in which she had
spent many years, was equally positive about the value of the
change. In a ward where the living space was shared with male
patients, she talked about the men who behaved like perfect
gentlemen, never failed to offer her a seat, etc. The activity
programme, meal-times and social periods were all livelier and
more enjoyable.

An important by-product appeared to be the blurring of roles
at the staff level. It was at this time the POTs (Patient Occupational Therapists) and PANs (Patient Assistant Nurses) flour-
ished. Both groups were led by trained people, the former by
an occupational therapist and the latter by a charge nurse. Patients
found themselves assisting staff members in bringing about a
vastly extended activity programme for the more dependent
patients.

During this stage of our development at the end of 1965, we
were preoccupied with dividing the hospital population on the
basis of function rather than geographically. At this time we
found many advantages in grouping patients according to their
similar needs. Geographical structuring later held strong appeal
and resulted in Dingleton eventually dividing its catchment area
into three separate county units and converting to a geographic
organization within the hospital.

New admissions presented no particular problem from the point
of view of finding placements in activities, because they generally had a short stay in hospital and resumed their outside work
and activities. The long-stay population had been relatively in-
active for years, but we found that with the growing strength
of the work therapy department we were creating work for
patients which had significance for the hospital community as a
whole. We did not follow the common trend at that time of having
people working for profit through subcontracted work for outside firms. We preferred to have them 'running their own hospital' as far as this was practicable, and focused on the interaction
within the work situation rather than on the financial rewards.
Even so, pay for work done was established, which meant that
virtually all the patients had money to spend. But our emphasis
on the general social skills involved in being in a work situation
had priority over 'learning to be a productive and efficient
worker'. To this end work therapists supervised groups of up to
twenty patients in programmes to do with serving in the canteen, waiting at tables, doing the housekeeping throughout the
hospital, working in the laundry and helping as POTs and PANs.
In addition, the young activity assistants worked in the geriatric

wards helping to find some way of interesting even the most organically deteriorated patients with music and movement, community singing, reading to the blind, and so on. The emphasis at this time was on functional roles for patients.

EXTRAMURAL DEVELOPMENTS

At the beginning of 1965 we started our first ex-patient club in the nearby town of Galashiels. This was followed by the establishment of a hostel for eight male patients on the hospital grounds. These patients all had outside employment and it was hoped that they would seek accommodation in the outside community once they had become established in their work setting. In June we began our first out-patient clinic in the nearby town of Hawick. Prior to this time out-patients had come to Dingleton. Although fairly centrally situated within its catchment area, it nevertheless entailed very difficult travelling for many patients and their relatives who had to use public transport.

We continued to respond to every invitation to visit outside organizations, such as rotary clubs, rural institutes, factories, schools, and so on. In January we had a meeting with the foremen at one of the large tweed mills. Before an audience of about fifty, we involved some of the employees in a socio-drama based on the admission of a new patient to Dingleton. In all our educational contacts with the outside community we tried, as far as possible, to start with a concrete situation and then moved gradually into the abstract ideas of psychiatry. If some of the local people were willing to volunteer to participate in a socio-drama, involvement by their peers became very much easier, and one could then hope to initiate a learning process.

In December we started a monthly meeting among family doctors, ministers and ourselves. It was felt that co-operative education by people playing a responsible role in the community would be valuable, and this proved to be the case. The two most important developments were the establishment of a Border Forum, and a Consultative Committee for the Co-ordination of Mental Health Services in the Borders. The latter was initiated after many preparatory discussions in September 1965. It was a formally constituted body involving the local authorities from the four counties which we served with representation from the general practitioners and from the staff at Dingleton. This body met quarterly and was immensely valuable in bringing about some degree of integration of services in the mental health field. The development of this organization is followed later in this book, but it is worth mentioning here that it evolved to form the Borders Health and Social Service Consultative Committee. This body included the general hospital and attempted to achieve the total integration of health services in this part of Scotland.

The Border Forum was a less formalized endeavour, and was really an experiment in community education. As a result of

many meetings, informal dinner parties, etc., we managed to persuade a group of leading people in the Borders to assume responsibility for open meetings in the larger towns. Our original planning group included a civil servant (who was proud of his humble origin), a local peer, a famous textile designer, a director of one of the largest tweed mills, a minister, a headmaster, the local Member of Parliament and myself. At first we considered the possibility that the Forum might simply appear on Border television and stimulate discussion in the homes of people living in the Borders. We decided, however, that we would prefer to have personal contact with local citizens in public meeting places. Our goal was to accomplish interaction of an informal kind, involving people in discussion about problems affecting the lives of people living in this region. At one time the Borders had united to fight the common enemy in England, and our rather ambitious goal was to attempt to recapture this common identity after several centuries, and apply ourselves to social problems such as the care of the aged, modern education, etc. The first meeting was planned for January 1966 in Galashiels.

SUMMARY OF THE THIRD YEAR

Our skill and confidence in developing and learning from living-learning or crisis situations, both aspects of social learning and growth, allowed us to involve wider parameters (Jones and Polak, 1968). In this chapter the satisfactory resolution of a problem relating to the Board of Management is described. Also, the hospital, represented by both the Board of Management and myself, faced the wrath of our employers, the South-Eastern Scotland Regional Hospital Board, in relation to our launching the activity assistant scheme without their approval. We could hardly tell them the truth – that we knew beforehand that they would disapprove and so had failed to inform them! The reason behind our conscious 'delinquency' was that an already established and successful programme is much more difficult to disallow than one on paper. At Henderson Hospital in London I had learned that growth might well entail the risk of putting one's job in jeopardy But there I lacked sanctions from above, where the Henderson Board of Management were my accusers. We were challenging the mores of mental health by treating psychopaths as potentially responsible adults, and delegating much of the responsibility for their management and 'treatment' to their own peer group. Three committees failed to liquidate our vulnerable project, thanks to the powerful support we received from Parliament and the press.

Now the circumstances were very different. We had an understanding and supportive Board of Management, and we went into battle as a united body against our employers. Here was a distant controlling bureaucracy who were prepared to judge before hearing the evidence. We had a cause worth fighting for, a scheme to better the quality and numbers for nurse recruitment

as the shortage of psychiatric nurses was a serious problem in
Scotland at that time; and we knew that if necessary we could
expose the Regional Board's closed-mindedness to the press.
This was never made explicit, and would have created bitter
feelings and no social learning would have occurred if we had
been forced to do so. Instead we involved the Board's own
bosses, the Home and Health Department for Scotland. We learned
a great deal from this painful confrontation which was finally
resolved in our favour! First, always choose your battleground
on an issue worth fighting for, even though it may cost your
job. When you are confronted, counter-attack so that the 'enemy'
is taken by surprise, not having realized that they may become
the victim. To do this at a later date gives the opposition ample
time to counter-attack and exploit their superior power. Finally,
one must believe in the basic decency of mankind, and in the
UK I never failed to get fair play from the highest authorities
in the land. In retrospect, with the steady growth of bureaucracy and the increasing difficulty in making direct contact with
the ultimate authority, it probably would have been more difficult
and time-consuming to confront the powers that be in 1981 than
in 1965. In addition, it may call for a new category of consumer
advocate with psychodynamic managerial and political skills, who
can expose the vulnerability of a powerful bureaucracy. Nevertheless, I still believe that therapeutic community principles and
decentralization translated into the educational, political, business and religious spheres offers a point of departure and a
methodology for those people hoping to break the oppressive
bonds of bureaucratic conformity.

Our use of living-learning situations within the hospital also
grew in frequency and effectiveness. A neutral facilitator from
an uninvolved area of the hospital chosen by both parties at risk
was invoked with increasing frequency. The culture of the hospital was changing and we were re-examining our priorities.
Thus the need for immediate involvement in a crisis situation
necessitated a flexible social organization. As an extreme
example, a serious crisis in the admission ward resulted in the
parties involved (patients and staff) agreeing that they wanted
me to act as facilitator. I was found participating in a Board of
Management meeting but left the board meeting immediately,
briefly explaining to the board members the need for expediency!
It seemed that the growth of what might be called a therapeutic
culture emanated from our day-to-day hospital practice, and by
contagion affected the hospital management committee's view of
their function. Our handling of problems outside the hospital
and even with the Regional Board in Edinburgh also showed how
a change in our approach to problem-solving inevitably affected
the environment so that change was made possible. This theme
develops further in later years.

Training and treatment became complementary and overlapped.
Thus even a Board of Management meeting had a training dimension, for example the concept of a hidden agenda became recog-

nized and covert emotional issues had to become overt and resolved if possible, if sound managerial decisions were to be made. Staff meetings, sensitivity training groups, community ward meetings involving all patients and staff were universal; and social forces in the environment of the hospital and outside were beginning to be a part of our concept of social organization and growth. Even the student nurses became aware of their identity and guarded their rights as a group as demonstrated by the incident when I tried to bring visitors to their sensitivity training group without first seeking their permission.

Inevitably some of this 'openness' and confidence in expressing feelings without fear of reprisal affected the patients' world. Not only were they gaining self-esteem by playing more responsible roles, but they were beginning to admit us into some of their more private and covert activities, as evidenced by the incident of the 'smoking corridor'. To have some awareness of the private world of the chronic schizophrenic was a new experience for some of us, and was a measure of a growing trust between patients and staff. (This whole subject was explored by a social anthropologist who chose to play the role of a patient at the Yale Psychiatric Institute and was accepted as such by the patients (Caudill, 1958).)

We were becoming increasingly aware of the importance of the role of the patient, even those who were severely handicapped. In addition to paid work in the dining halls as waitresses, etc., in the wards as cleaners, in the laundry, garden, piggery, etc., we developed the POTs and PANs, each group under the supervision of a staff member. The POTs made activity programmes available to the more chronic wards and the PANs helped with meal-times and other chores for relatively helpless geriatric patients. These activities, including the entire staffing of the canteen by patients, meant that they were contributing to the life of the hospital and became increasingly identified with it.

Linked with this functional development we 'exploited' the social environment of the hospital to stimulate activity and positive interaction. As already mentioned, the physical structure of the hospital was greatly improved, and a new canteen and social centre, shared by both patients and staff, was opened. We also reorganized the hospital to bring about a closer integration of the sexes, but only after lengthy discussions with the patients. At this point in time we were more concerned with the development of functional stratification of patients within the hospital than dividing them into geographical units representing their county domicile – which did occur later.

Finally, the third year saw the establishment of our first ex-patient club in a nearby town, an out-patient clinic in another town, and a hostel within the hospital grounds for eight male patients, all of whom had outside employment. Our infiltration into the outside environment concerning prevention, after-care and mental health education was also gaining momentum. We began a monthly meeting interacting with family doctors and

ministers and discussed matters of common interest, for example the dying patient, incest, etc.

At a more formal level a Consultative Committee for the Co-ordination of Mental Health Service in the Borders was started and met every three months until my departure four years later. This opened up communication and co-operation among the family doctors, the local authorities of the three counties we served, and ourselves.

As already described, the Border Forum was established where leaders in Border society agreed to meet in public halls and interact with the general public on matters pertaining to mental health. The plan was to choose a topic of general interest and then have the panel start a discussion with a view to 'warming up' the audience. I was to act as facilitator and invoke audience participation.

I think it is important to note that the process of reaching out to the community, through the establishment of such organiz-ations as the Border Forum, the Consultative Committee for Co-ordination of Health Services, etc., was enhanced by social interaction in whatever setting seemed appropriate and natural to the culture, for example dining parties in my own home, some staff met and interacted in the local pub, etc. The culture in Dingleton that emerged was one that blurred the roles of work and play, or one's work and one's social and leisure activities. For me that is the key to enjoying life: blurring this work/play dichotomy so that what is work is fun, exciting and challenging 'play', and an integrated part of one's life.

This chapter has focused on areas where historically change in hospital practice was most marked, all of which reflected on the life of the patient. We are talking about a time sixteen years ago when social psychiatry in the USA was in its infancy. The late President Kennedy in a Congressional Committee in 1963 stated (US President, 1963):

> I propose a national mental health program to assist in the inauguration of a wholly new emphasis and approach to care for the mentally ill. Governments at every level - federal, state, and local, private foundations, and individual citizens - must all face up to their responsibilities in this area.

This was the start of the community mental health programme in the USA. It began somewhat abruptly with huge federal funding, and was not the result of a slow evolution of social psychiatry after the Second World War as in Britain. In order to keep some perspective it is also appropriate to point out that changes in social psychiatry of the order and extent of Dingleton were to be found nowhere else in Britain at this time. We were, however, influencing psychiatry in other areas of the world and linking up with considerable developments in social psychiatry in Holland and Scandinavia at or even before that time.

The fourth year, 1966:
decentralization of the system begins

INTRODUCTION

The year 1966 was to see many changes due to the coming and
going of staff. More important organizationally was a continued
trend toward a more integrated team structure. The previous
year had seen a move to integrate the sexes on the patient wards
along with a very pleasant large social centre and canteen open
to both patients and staff.

Although it had been divided into the usual wards for new
admissions, geriatrics, etc., until now the hospital had been
largely responsible to one hospital central authority, that is
the Senior Staff Committee. Six years earlier when visiting the
USA I had become friendly with and visited Dr Leonardo Garcia
(1960) at Clarinda State Hospital in Iowa. His decentralization of
a large state hospital into separate geographical units serving
separate counties had made a deep impression on me.

We were not yet ready to form separate county units with
their own staffs, but a start was made in this direction by making the three senior psychiatrists leaders of three staff teams
in anticipation of later redistribution of patients into three
separate county units. This meant that at this time patients were
still residents in 'functional' units according to their clinical
needs. Within those units they were divided up according to
which psychiatrist (and his team) looked after them. This evolutionary process was completed a year later with the emergence
of separate county units in 1967.

Interpersonal staff conflicts lessened during the year due to
several factors. In the first case the two most controversial
figures, Matron and Dr Small, both retired and were replaced
by people who chose to work at Dingleton because of its growing
reputation as an open system relatively free from the abuse of
authority. (This factor always seemed to be a major attraction
in recruitment and the numbers of applicants steadily grew for
all categories of staff.) Second, the numbers and quality of
trained staff were growing and we reached six doctors and six
social workers for the first time; in addition, the top nursing
administration grew from two in Matron's time to four during
1966. Third, the concept and practice of multiple leadership in
a multidisciplinary setting was growing. Dividing staff into
three separate clinical teams resulted in more integrated practice,
improved communication, information-sharing and shared
decision-making. But the Senior Staff Committee now met daily

to insure that the hospital identity took precedence over the emerging team identity and the strengthened professional identities.

Finally, the role of a facilitator in areas of conflict became an integral part of our use of social learning (Jones 1976b). A facilitator was a person acceptable to both sides of any interpersonal conflict chosen for his objectivity and knowledge of group process and dynamics. The aim was to facilitate the process of social learning.

INTRAMURAL DEVELOPMENTS

Staff changes
This year staff changes contributed to the efficiency of the hospital and its social structure. Late in the year, a number of resignations and retirements coincided with the structural changes we had planned and discussed for months. This fortuitous combination of events made the transitions much smoother.

In the first part of 1966 our Matron left to be replaced by her deputy, Michael Clark. Unlike his predecessor, Michael communicated freely with his peers and greatly strengthened the senior nursing staff by having a Deputy Principal Nursing Officer (DPNO) as well as three Assistant Principal Nursing Officers (APNO). This solid group at the top of the nursing hierarchy provided a very valuable stabilizing influence on the whole hospital, although I was constantly on guard against Michael's tendency to prefer the administrative to the clinical role.

Paul Polak, an experienced psychiatrist who came to us in 1965 from Fort Logan Mental Health Center, Denver, Colorado, returned to Colorado. He was an immensely active and imaginative psychiatrist who was keenly aware of the need to link the intra- and extramural dimensions, and whose crisis-intervention policy stimulated us to much greater involvement in the community. Lindsay Madew, who had done a fine job in Australia in the rehabilitation of long-stay patients, replaced him.

My deputy, Dr Ken Morrice, left to spend a year at Fort Logan, where he further enhanced his reputation as one of the best social psychiatrists in the two countries. He was replaced by Jim Todd who had been a Senior Registrar at the University Clinic in Aberdeen. Perhaps most significant of all, Dr Small, who had been on the staff for many years, retired. Two experienced social workers joined our staff. Joy Tuxford, who had worked with me for five years at the original therapeutic community at Henderson Hospital, took up a research post. David Anderson was made the chief social worker with the special task of developing community psychiatry.

Structural changes
Multiple leadership began to emerge as early as 1964 (Jones,
1968a, pp. 33-42). By now instead of having disagreements with
my senior colleagues or with the Matron it became increasingly
possible to have discussion with neutral, uninvolved leadership
emerging and playing the role which we came to refer to as a
facilitator. Any disagreement could usually be turned into a
learning situation.

Early in the year we agreed to develop smaller more integrated
clinical units rather than one large hospital staff. We decided to
try a preliminary division of the hospital staff into three units,
each led by one of the three senior doctors. Thus the functional
social organization of the hospital described in the last chapter
gave way to smaller more integrated units.

This rearrangement of staff did not affect the patients themselves, but was only concerned with tightening up the integration
of staff into three separate units. This anticipated by over a
year the much more important division of the hospital into three
separate county teams as described in the next chapter. As a
start in the process of decentralization, we decided that each of
the three major counties to be served by Dingleton would have
a senior and a junior psychiatrist, two social workers (one
qualified PSW and one unqualified), one Assistant Principal
Nursing Officer and later in the year a secretary was added.
The advantages of such a plan were obvious. The team members
were concerned with a distinct geographical area; instead of having to get to know all 68 family doctors in the Borders and other
personnel, they now had to concern themselves only with the
doctors and local authority personnel in their particular county.
By the same token, personnel concerned with mental health in
the county knew with whom to deal on the Dingleton staff.

The six doctors now appeared only once or twice a week at
the admission ward meetings and thus were free to do more work
on the long-stay, geriatric wards and in the community. Moreover, the fact that the three county teams had their own separate
patient population in the admission wards meant that they could
become more effective in the handling of the treatment requirements of individual cases. Thus, one county began to meet with
their own patients in a smaller subgroup, and this applied to
family groups, individual interviews, and so on. In this way we
saw a much greater flexibility in the treatment programme than
had been apparent in the past.

A complicating factor at this time was the retirement of Dr
Small and her replacement by Dr Jean Smith. We had known for
a long time that many of the referrals to Dingleton had come
through Dr Small by family doctors who approached her at night
by telephone, and she had admitted people by 'the back door'.
Now that referrals were being made to the county teams we had
much more opportunity to scrutinize admissions either by doing
home or domiciliary visits or by an admission evaluation session
at the hospital. This resulted in fewer admissions and consider-

ably more domiciliary work. In fact, community psychiatry was growing, each county team vying with the others in trying to develop close contacts with the family doctors and local authorities in their areas.

Another by-product of the recent change and rethinking about patient care was the establishment of a unit for mentally retarded patients. Glenkinnon became such a ward and brought together all the male and female mentally retarded residents at Dingleton, a total of forty patients. The immediate result of this change was a rather inert and depressing group. However, this acted as a stimulus and we contacted family doctors and others to see if there were backward people in the community who could profitably come in as day patients. We also tried to see if there were retired people in the neighbourhood community who had skills to share, such as joinery, to an active programme for these people. The patients on this ward began to make small articles to sell in the canteen, and these activity groups seemed to be quite a success. The morale in Glenkinnon became surprisingly high. Some months after the establishment of Glenkinnon Ward we paid a visit to Gogarburn Mental Deficiency Hospital in Edinburgh, mainly to discuss policy. They were perfectly happy about sending us mentally retarded patients who would benefit from living in the Borders close to their families. A possible exchange scheme was discussed as was the desirability of having some day patients on Glenkinnon.

Eden Ward for disturbed long-stay patients of both sexes had come under the charge of Dr Lindsay Madew. It became a rehabilitation ward which tried to bring about a more rapid return of patients to the community. Lindsay felt that patients should be sent back to the community whenever possible. I agreed with this in principle, but feared that the pendulum might swing too far, and that we might initially overwhelm the community. This might do a dis-service both to the patients and to the families or people with whom they lived. Later that year the Selkirkshire team divided the large Eden Ward group of 77 patients into two smaller groups: one where the orientation was toward the community, and the other toward an adjustment to life in Dingleton. In this context there was a great deal of interest among all the doctors about the selection of people who were capable of achieving a higher quality of living within the hospital than outside. While retaining our effort to rehabilitate as many people as possible to the community, it was an important clinical challenge to distinguish the relative merits of rehabilitation to the outside from a relatively satisfying life in Dingleton. Put more simply, people who have repeatedly failed to make an adjustment outside have to be considered in terms of their role in hospital. How could we develop a varied and to some extent a self-supporting way of life for people living in hospital? This implied an evolutionary process toward a 'village settlement' and away from a traditional stereotyped hospital environment (Jones, 1979b).

There are other examples of such 'subcultures' in society; perhaps the largest and oldest are the various Roman Catholic religious orders. However, a Protestant society dislikes the idea of people being segregated from society, and there is a strong negative attitude toward the institutionalized patient. My point is that there is nothing wrong with institutionalization provided it creates for some individuals a better society than they would find in the ordinary community (Peele et al., 1977; Jones, 1979b); I have discussed elsewhere the therapeutic communities stemming from the Synanon model compared with the therapeutic community model described in this book (Jones, 1979c). One could say that vagrants are another example of a subculture of people who have established a way of life with its own characteristics and with the almost complete avoidance of a 'responsible' and financially rewarding way of life. Synanon in the USA exemplifies the same sort of thing for drug addicts. A significant feature of Synanon is that it is an organization which explicitly excludes professional workers. This may well be its strong point. Along with this is the fact that it makes, as far as I know, relatively little attempt to select patients who will respond to treatment, because there is no end to the treatment or rehabilitation programme as they see it (Jones, 1979c, p. 143). The hard core of vagrant chronic alcoholics may also represent a society apart. It may be that any attempt to bring them into a fairly orthodox social structure will fail, and that the only way in which a society can be built around them is to allow them to have living environments in which they develop their own way of life.

The admission ward had great difficulty in accommodating itself to the new three-county system, as it affected the staffing on their ward. This was understandable because, in theory at least, all six doctors shared the mixed male/female admission ward as did the other members of the county teams, particularly the social workers. In the past the admission ward had one doctor in charge of the male ward and another in charge of the female ward. This meant that the nursing staff's role relationship with the doctor was relatively simple and familiar. Now the nurses had to think of their patients in terms of the county plus the doctor to which they belonged and related. This meant that from a relatively simple ward culture the nurses now had a much more complex one involving many more people. In addition, there was beginning to become apparent an awareness of tugs in two directions: one toward a ward identity and one toward a team identity. The latter was not strong at this point. The nurses on the admission ward who had done some excellent pioneering work in developing a role for themselves in the community, following up ex-patients or doing home visits with a psychiatrist at the request of a family doctor, now began to feel their function was limited to the ward, and that the county teams were taking over the community work. Another trend was that the senior doctors began to feel the admission ward was so well covered by staff that they could focus on the long-stay and geriatric wards, and

in particular on their community involvement.

I presented a particular problem because I had a dual role: that of physician superintendent as well as consultant to the Berwickshire county team. This meant that for weeks I might be so heavily committed that I had very little contact with the admission ward or even with the Berwickshire team.

In November 1966, approximately a month after the start of one admission ward for the three county teams, I asked permission for Michael Clark, the Principal Nursing Officer, to come to the meeting of the admission ward staff. I knew it would be an important meeting in relation to the role of senior nurses in both hospital and community work. I quote from my diary notes:

> There appeared to be a problem with the role relationship between the ward nurses and the three Assistant Principal Nursing Officers who were assigned to each of the three county teams. Michael was annoyed and said I was getting on his back about the clinical and community involvement of senior nurses. Indeed this is true because Michael himself is staying completely out of clinical involvement and I am concerned about his role.
>
> Reg Elliott, one of the two charge nurses on the admission ward, came to the point by immediately launching into his feelings of anger. He said that since the three-county-team system had been initiated, the admission ward nurses had been bypassed and were doing practically no domiciliary visits. He saw this as directly attributable to the fact that the APNOs were attached to county teams whereas ward nurses were not. The matter of attaching ward nurses to teams had been discussed at length, and it had been decided that this could not be justified as there were not enough nurses. On further analysis it became difficult to understand exactly why the admission ward nurses were excluded from doing home visits and follow-up work generally. This seemed more in the realm of fantasy than of fact, and no one wanted Reg or anyone else to discontinue their extramural activities. It seemed much more likely that staff energy was occupied by the current disturbance which naturally accompanied the transition to a team system and by the anxieties of the nursing staff within the admission ward in forming new role relationships with the county-team members. The learning situation seems to be essentially around how the new social structure of the three county clinical teams interferes with function particularly on the admission ward and requires the establishment of new role relationships.

With the new social organization on the admission ward and the changing leadership, it was not clear where the power lay. I was a leader of a kind, but not the sort of clinical leader that Paul Polak and Ken Morrice had previously represented on their res-

pective male and female admission wards. It must have been clear
to most people that I was not competing for leadership in the
clinical sphere, but saw this as properly belonging to Lindsay
Madew and Jim Todd who had replaced Ken and Paul. As already
mentioned, Michael Clark, the Principal Nursing Officer, resisted
coming into the clinical setting. I felt that he unconsciously
sensed the impending power struggle and preferred to keep out
of it if possible.

At ward level the confusion and struggle to form new identities
and role relationships meant that the nurses felt somewhat de-
prived; they no longer held the key position with the ward doctors, but were in competition with the other doctors, social
workers and senior nurses from all three county teams.

At the regular weekly Journal Club seminar I read a paper
which discussed social structure in relation to hospitals. What
emerged in the discussion was a new awareness of the problems
of structure and function. We had taken weeks to elaborate a
plan for the new admission ward and its interrelationships with
the three county teams which represented a formulated social
organization. It now remained to be seen how it would function.
We realized that structure and function were complementary
and that each depended on the other. On this occasion we set up
a social structure and then waited to see how this would function
Usually at Dingleton we worked the other way round, allowing
people to find a function or place for themselves in the hospital
provided that this met the needs of the subunit they chose.
There were obvious limits concerning vacancies, fair distribution
etc., but largely the structure accommodated itself to the new
member. In the example of the new admission ward described
above, structure and function were helped to equilibrate, but
it was a slow and painful process. Our democratic planning process of discussing any proposed change in social structure with
everyone concerned was not yet fully established.

The formal responsibility for the hospital was invested in the
three 'administrators': the Principal Nursing Officer, the
Hospital Secretary and myself. This arrangement was imposed on
us from the start by our bureaucratic bosses in Edinburgh who
had little awareness, if any, of our democratic egalitarian social
structure. We met daily at 8.30 a.m. for half an hour and discussed administrative matters. If the topics concerned other
people, they were invited to attend. We then joined the Senior
Staff Committee for 45 minutes, where we fed back any deliber-
ations or suggestions to this executive staff body. In July 1966
we met at 8.30 a.m. with no other people present so we could be
more efficient, but extended the time of the SSC so that any
executive decision would be taken in conjunction with them. In
this way all important decisions were made by the Senior Staff
and the teams complemented one another rather than competed.

Delegation of authority and power
The early evolution of the decentralized programme represented
by the three county teams meant that I became less directly involved in many situations concerning decision-making at a
senior level. During one week I was in Edinburgh on three
occasions on essential business, had three evening speaking
engagements, and a home domiciliary visit in Berwickshire. I
felt I was losing touch with the hospital at a time when my two
senior colleagues were developing new ideas which they fed into
the SSC. In my absence they sometimes achieved a degree of
group acceptance which was difficult to modify, even if I had
wished to do so. We were much nearer to multiple leadership than
we had ever been. The leadership in the admission ward was
largely in the hands of two psychiatrists, Lindsay and Jim. The
decision-making machinery was less evident at the centre and
more apparent at the periphery. For example, it was quite explicit and minuted at the SSC that because of the pressure of
work on secretaries, the nurses' notes would in future be hand-
written. In my absence both these decisions by the SSC were
reversed and a reorganization of the secretaries resulted in
which each team had a secretary of its own. This reorganization
covered not only their typing requirements, but appointments,
typing of nurses' notes, and so on. This was a good plan, but
my secretary became associated with the Berwickshire team, and
I felt this was a further inroad on my function as the hospital
superintendent. This democratic SSC function was what we had
always worked toward and it was now actually happening. My
power was certainly lessened, and I felt this was a good thing
and in line with our philosophy, even if I did not always like it!

A unilateral decision and confrontation
It may be that as a reaction to this lessening of my authority I
made the only unilateral decision I can remember during my
employment at Dingleton. This was in connection with a newly
formed house committee for the nurses' residence, consisting of
an International Voluntary Service student, a Norwegian social
worker and a nurse who was a work therapist in the canteen.
These three were elected to be the House Committee and asked
me to approve a number of proposals about freedom of resident
staff at night. These included the use of the staff coffee room
without any time limit, and the opening of the sitting-room both
in the male and female nurses' homes. These reforms were long
overdue, but in view of the fact that, of these three people,
two were temporary staff and the nurse planned to live outside
the hospital, my response - without consulting anyone, - was
that I was not prepared to accept their recommendations without
further enquiry. I insisted on a meeting with some senior staff
and all the resident staff to see if they endorsed the recommendations of this small committee. I felt that in view of the difficulties we had experienced in the past over residents' behaviour,
we could not sanction this degree of freedom unless every resi-

dent was prepared to assume some responsibility for the new scheme.

During the discussion of this incident at the SSC both Jimmy Millar and Michael Clark said that I had, in fact, not made a unilateral decision, but simply insisted on a meeting so that the rights of everyone concerned could be heard. A meeting among the Principal Nursing Officer, Hospital Secretary, myself and the resident staff was arranged. At this meeting it appeared that a number of the resident staff knew nothing about the house committee which was openly discredited, and the decision was taken to form a new and more representative house committee involving some of the long-term residents and not just a few temporary staff. The new house committee made its wishes known to the SSC and their recommendations were adopted. These were similar to the original proposals, but now reflected the views of everyone concerned.

EXTRAMURAL DEVELOPMENTS

Mental Health Consultative Committee
In the first quarter of 1966 I noted:

> There are distinct possibilities of developments in the com-
> munity field that could make Dingleton as effective a thera-
> peutic community extramurally as I hope it is intramurally. On
> Monday we had the third meeting of the Mental Health Con-
> sultative Committee for the Borders. This brings together the
> local authorities, family doctors and hospital authorities of the
> Borders. Dr Brodie, the Superintendent of Peel Hospital [the
> Borders' general hospital], has been co-opted; he spoke quite
> frankly about the possibility of having a combined health
> centre with Dingleton and the local authorities, and that the
> new projected Peel Hospital might well be built near Dingleton.
> [This in fact did ultimately take place but the actual building
> was delayed for fourteen years!] The advent of the new plan
> for the development of the Borders and the appointment of
> Johnston Marshall, Professor of Town and Country Planning at
> Edinburgh University, as the new consultant to the Borders
> Development Plan, should all make for a favourable climate.

> In September we had our fifth meeting of the Consultative
> Committee for the Co-ordination of the Mental Health Services.
> The inevitable difficulty of integrating organizations under
> different managements became evident. The hospital personnel
> and the family doctors seemed to agree fairly well, but rivalries
> developed between the three Medical Officers of Health and their
> respective county clerks from the three counties which we
> served. The county clerks complained that, because they had
> not been properly briefed about what was going on and because
> we were moving far too rapidly, they had no time to consult

with their respective county local authority committees. It was
pointed out that this committee had no formal power and that
progress toward informal co-ordination on a goodwill basis was
our modest goal.

To set an example of co-operation with the other agencies,
Dingleton agreed to making available our three psychiatric social
workers on a joint-user basis with the local authorities. This
meant that, with our three PSWs and the one already employed
by the local authorities, we had four people who could share the
community work in the Borders for the mutual benefit of all the
health agencies.

Psychiatric social work
In line with these developments was the question of the future
of our own social work department, and the role of the senior
social worker, David Anderson. He had joined us more than a
year previously with a special assignment to develop community
work. However, he seemed still to be getting too involved intramurally and to have too little interest in the extramural dimension.
Although our infiltration into the community was progressing
satisfactorily it was essentially an extension of our intramural
work. I had hoped that David would act as a leader-catalyst
and link up creatively with the latent mental health resources
in the community. This he did later, but at this time he apparently felt more secure in the established culture within Dingleton
and could not yet see how to create a therapeutic community
model in our catchment area. The social workers did home visits,
consultations with family doctors, etc., but as yet had no particular identity as community workers.

Positive sanctions from the central authority
In April I had an opportunity to talk with Dr Brotherston, the
Chief Medical Officer for Scotland. He was very interested in
the plan for an integrated health service in the Borders. He
indicated that he would be glad to give active support to any
plan that we cared to put forward.

I talked to him about the possibility of Dingleton becoming a
social resource rather than a psychiatric hospital, that its
function might well change to that of a temporary haven for
people in need, irrespective of their clinical diagnosis. This
would have fitted in with the changing emphasis in psychiatry
in which clinical work was begun at the earliest possible moment
and kept as far as practicable within the community.

Family doctors
In July 1966 I attended a meeting of the Local Medical Committee
of the Border counties at Ednam House, Kelso. The Medical
Officer of Health for the counties of Roxburgh and Selkirk had
written a letter at our request, outlining the need for medical
reports from Dingleton to his colleagues when there was the
likelihood of some follow-through action by the local authority.

This gave me the opportunity to explain the developments which
were being realized mainly through the work of the Borders
Mental Health Co-ordination Committee. From my weekly diary
notes a description of this meeting is as follows:

> Approximately ten family doctors were at the Local Medical
> Committee meeting, and they showed a great deal of interest
> in what was developing. I went on to say we intended to
> raise at the next meeting of the Co-ordination Committee the
> possibility of a joint-user arrangement with our three psychi-
> atric social workers and Iris Short, the local authority's social
> worker. Through co-ordination all four might be employed
> and paid equally by the local authority and by the National
> Health Service. Dr Sproule, one of the general practitioners,
> was able to say how much he appreciated having the help of
> Betty Ashby, one of our social workers, without having
> actually to contact a psychiatrist. Other doctors said they
> found this a very desirable change in the structure of the
> mental health services because they had many social problems
> they wanted help with rather than a psychiatric opinion. I
> also mentioned the plan for partial decentralization at Dingleto
> into county units which would help the integration of mental
> health services. Finally, I touched on Joy Tuxford's
> community-attitude research which meant they would all have
> the opportunity for an interview with her and could express
> their views about Dingleton and the psychiatric services
> generally.
>
> As the climate was so favourable, I asked if they would
> agree to having copies of the discharge letter, which they
> received from us when a patient left hospital, sent to the
> Medical Officer of Health or his local authority personnel
> when this seemed appropriate. To my amazement there was
> general agreement that this would be a good plan provided,
> of course, the patient had given his consent and the family
> doctor was also contacted by the social worker to obtain his
> permission. I asked if I could be given assurance that this
> decision would be binding for all 68 family doctors in the
> Borders, and was told the Local Medical Committee had this
> power. We felt it would be advisable for the Medical Officers
> of Health to circulate reports describing our meeting to the
> doctors in their counties so that any doctors who disapproved
> would make this known.
>
> The question of domiciliary home visits raised mixed feeling
> and criticism was directed, I think properly, at the involve-
> ment of too many people in the county teams from Dingleton.
> We had ourselves experienced the adverse effect on some
> Berwickshire patients of too large a team converging on an
> unsuspecting patient. It was thought that the matter should
> be discussed at the time when the doctor rang up requesting
> a domiciliary visit, and after deciding on the appropriate team
> the family doctor could prepare the patient for such a contin-

gency. The family doctor invariably accompanies the team and introduces them to his patient. There seemed to be preference for sending the patient with his or her relative to Dingleton for assessment. There was no indication that the doctors themselves could find the time to accompany the patient to hospital. It was generally agreed that a real emergency must be treated as such and the patient admitted to hospital without delay. The family doctors were not keen on the nurse ringing up the day a patient is discharged from hospital to inform them of the medication the patient is receiving. They preferred the psychiatrist to do this so they could question him if they wanted. They were unanimous in wanting a written report for their files; and were also unanimous in accepting the fact that Dr Jean Smith might act as my deputy; in fact, they seemed to relish the idea!

uture geriatrician

ontinuing development of our community involvement made it .ear that if we were going to make the most of the services .ready existing for geriatric care we would need a full-time eriatrician. Such a person would be able to integrate the .cilities available from the point of view of general medicine, sychiatry and the local authority. We already had two reports .n the subject, one from the Superintendent of Peel Hospital .nd the other from Iris Short, the social worker shared by the .cal authorities and ourselves. It looked as though we had .ough beds for old people provided the service was well organ-.ed and beds were properly used. Dr Brodie from Peel Hospital, .is Short and myself discussed the whole matter with the .egional Board and received every encouragement to continue .ur plans for an integrated service headed by a geriatric .onsultant.

UMMARY OF THE FOURTH YEAR

.ur growing preference for domiciliary visits, preferably .companied by the family doctor, met with strong resistance. .r Small, before her retirement, had allowed the general prac-.tioners to use Dingleton more or less as they liked, which .ten meant removing troublesome cases from their homes to the .spital with the clinical assessment occurring after admission. .w we screened patients in their homes which meant more work .I around, but involved the families from the start and allowed . to assess the strengths and weaknesses in the family for .ture reference. Needless to say, many patients who previously .d slipped into hospital with Dr Small's connivance were now .le to stay in the outside community where a treatment and .pport programme invoking community resources in collaboration .th ourselves was accomplished. The emergence of the three county teams meant that a team

comprising a psychiatrist, social worker and nurse did the
initial work outside the hospital, leaving the majority of staff in
the hospital to carry on as usual. (The patients were not yet
subdivided in county units according to their county of origin;
this came later.) New roles tended to be seen as more exciting
and a good deal of rivalry between the old (the hospital) and th
new (the community) roles emerged. Despite prolonged discussion, this issue was never fully resolved. Another by-produ
of the county-team system was a tendency for the county-team
identity to transcend the hospital identity. This discussion continued until I left, but we became aware of the dangers of such
splitting. Competition for staff, money, physical facilities, etc.
had to be matched against the overall hospital needs. For this
to happen the SSC, which included members of all three teams,
had to be kept informed of all major issues throughout the hospital system. Only then could a fair distribution of resources be
accomplished and cross-fertilization of ideas emerge. This
amounted to a hierarchy of identities: hospital, county teams
and professional discipline, in that order. Without such a sensible evolution we would soon have faced the horrors of 'territo
iality' so familiar and so destructive in the present-day scene.

We continued our role as leaders in the community in an
attempt to achieve an integrated health plan for the Borders.
The newly formed Mental Health Consultative Committee met
every three months, but inevitably it became clear that local
authorities, family doctors and hospital personnel had very
different frames of reference. Our basic concepts of two-way
communication, shared decision-making and social learning were
largely unfamiliar to the other organizations. Here lies one of
the basic problems of bureaucracy. The centralization of power
with the resulting increase in the number of bureaucrats and
the distance from the consumer, all conspire to create a false
image at the top. Flooded by issues which are inevitably dis-
torted by communication through several layers of the bureaucracy, the central authority makes its decisions. In the absence
of two-way communication or feedback it learns nothing from its
mistakes. To make matters worse, the central authority almost
always chooses to communicate with 'the' hospital administrator
If the hospital is run on traditional hierarchical lines, then wha
has been described above has also occurred in the intra-hospit
communication system. Imagine what a patient or junior staff
member's complaint, if 'important' enough to enter the pipeline
sounds like when it reaches the top regional authority; or put
reverse, what quality of reply does he eventually receive, if
any!

Despite the relatively simple administrative system in the
Borders, involving only 100,000 people, we never achieved a
truly democratic or open system within the Mental Health Consultative Committee or its later more extensive counterpart. Bu
as a hospital group our impact on the Borders community was
considerable.

Perhaps the outstanding feature of 1966 was the flexibility of
the hospital system as manifested by our willingness to change
along the lines of organizational development (Jones, 1976a,
pp. 8-15). The dynamics of an open system with its shared
leadership, information-sharing, interaction, discussion, social
learning, decision-making by consensus and constant re-
evaluation lead inevitably to a process of change. Not only was
the social organization of the hospital in a state of constant flux,
but we were deploying increasing resources into the community
linking up with the local family doctors, starting community
clinics, and involving the school system, etc. Nor were we limiting ourselves to a medical (treatment) role. Education of the
general public (Border Forum), prevention (infiltration into the
school system), integration with local politics (Mental Health
Consultative Committee) and integration with the Home and
Health Department in Edinburgh (Dr John Brotherston, Chief
Medical Officer for Scotland) were all part of this growth process.

Chapter 5

The fifth year, 1967:
decentralization into three county units

INTRODUCTION

The two outstanding trends in 1966 had been: (a) the organizational development of the hospital, resulting from a flexible
social structure and evolution toward a largely decentralized
hospital; and (b) the increasing quantity and quality of trained
staff. These trends continued, resulting in three county units
for both patients and staff. The total separation of the hospital
into three semi-autonomous units based on their geographical
identity was not fully realized. Our total patient population of
400 patients did not make it practicable to have three separate
admission units with their inevitable drain on staff. The same
applied to the special unit for the mentally retarded. So we
ended up with a mixture of geographical and functional hospital
units.

Recruitment also continued to improve. This was made possible
by a supportive Hospital Management Committee and the great
administrative skills of Jimmy Millar, who somehow managed to
convince the authorities of the Regional Board in Edinburgh to
increase our financial support. Such political and administrative
gains would probably be more difficult in our present-day
bureaucracies where communication and discussion at an interpersonal level between hospital and the higher authorities is
blocked by the several layers of bureaucracy. We had a direct
communication network from every part of our hospital system to
the daily meeting of the Senior Staff Committee; thence through
Jimmy Millar to our Board of Management, who almost always
understood our needs, and sanctioned his further approach to
the ultimate authority in Edinburgh. Open systems make a
strong case against large systems of centralized power with
their 'invisible' authority at the top and their impersonal and
often disinterested interactions all too common today!

RECRUITMENT OF STAFF

As in the previous year the numbers and quality of staff showed
a steady improvement. It was during this year that we achieved
seven doctors: six psychiatrists, three of whom were fully
trained, plus three residents or registrars, and a seventh doctor with the grading of Senior House Officer who was primarily
concerned with the health of the old people. When I started at

Dingleton we had three senior doctors, one registrar and a
Senior House Officer. The nursing staff also was growing both
in quality and quantity, and included Michael Clark, the
Principal Nursing Officer (PNO); a deputy; and three Assistant
Principal Nursing Officers (APNOs); and the Nursing Tutor.
This meant that there were six experienced and competent
nurses all skilled in administrative, clinical and teaching roles.
In addition, our three-year nurse-training programme for
student nurses, a two-year programme for pupil nurses, a one-
year programme for post-registration nurses who had completed
their general training, and a one-year advanced course for
nurses represented a great improvement compared with previous
years. From a total of seven nurses in training five years ago,
we now had fifty. The social work department, too, had risen
from one psychiatric social worker to five trained social workers.
During this year I felt we had achieved approximately six leaders
from the fields of nursing administration, research, social work
and medicine. We had, in fact, achieved multiple leadership in a
multidisciplinary setting (Jones, 1968a, pp. 33-42).

Along with this increase in strength and experience there was,
I think, a growing awareness of our limitations. We had been
perhaps too intent on developing the therapeutic community concept with its emphasis on social organization, roles, role relationships and interaction generally. We began to listen to students
from nursing, medicine and social work questioning the adequacy
of the training they were getting. We were reminded of our
tendency to devalue formal training and teaching of the more
orthodox kind. Possibly we had become too preoccupied with
learning as a social process for the needs of some trainees.

INTRAMURAL DEVELOPMENTS

Nurse status increases
The doctors, and certainly the senior doctors, stopped playing
the leadership role in the admission wards' patient-staff meetings. This came about gradually. To begin with, one of the
three senior doctors felt a greater obligation to spend his time
in Eden Ward for long-stay patients, which he felt needed him
much more than the admission ward. Another factor was that
Dr Raschild, who came occasionally to the admission wards'
meetings, clashed badly with the male charge nurse, Reg.
Finally, Reg said at one of the Wednesday staff meetings on the
admission ward that in his opinion it would be better if the
doctors did not come at all and left the ward meeting to the
nurses. He chose to ignore the fact that the psychiatrists had a
much longer training than nurses and were an essential part of
our teaching programme. However, it was agreed that the charge
nurses represented the continuity in treatment and might well
be the best people to lead the daily ward treatment groups. Reg
pointed out that the junior nurses would find it easier to partici-

pate if doctors were not there, but the underlying agenda was that the nurses simply needed a vote of confidence in their ability to handle the day-to-day problems of the ward themselves I agreed in principle, provided Michael Clark, the Principal Nursing Officer, and the Assistant Principal Nursing Officers participated regularly so that any interpersonal conflict with a patient or staff member would be dealt with in a relatively objective way.

It seemed desirable to get Michael Clark more involved clinicall so that he might become a leader and teacher in group work on a par with the psychiatrist. Moreover, this fitted in with our developing plans for a one-year training programme for four specially selected nurses as clinical specialists. This programme, which we shared with Edinburgh University, seemed almost certain to materialize. We had two meetings with Professor Morris Carstairs, Dr Henry Walton and Miss Bruce, the matron of the Royal Edinburgh Hospital, and we hoped that the programme would begin in October with four nurses spending six months at Edinburgh, followed by six months with us. If Michael Clark and his senior nurses were to be prepared for such an important test of their training skills, then they had to be much more clinically involved. I did not see this as giving in to Reg's somewhat aggressive aspirations, but felt it was an evolution toward a mor independent nursing role, complementing the psychiatrist in the clinical field. It was agreed that in the first instance, to relieve the doctors' anxieties, it would be desirable for them to observe through the one-way screen and participate in the review session after the ward meeting. On the whole the doctors felt that they would be glad to have time to devote to the long-stay wards, and particularly to community psychiatry which was making increasing demands on their time.

Training of senior nurses
From the previous developments followed concern about the clinical and group work training of the six senior nurses. The three APNOs were relatively new, and the Nurse Tutor had experienced no formal training in groups. With a view to improving this situation and further integrating medical and nursing work, it was suggested that the doctors' meeting on Mondays at noon should include the six senior nurses. It was felt that at this meeting we should talk more about feelings, with a view to training and resolution of interpersonal conflicts. As always, this 'agenda' was on a trial basis and if it seemed unproductive would be replaced.

Student nurses sensitivity training
The weekly meeting with the student nurses at three o'clock on Mondays was facilitated by the Nurse Tutor and myself, with no other senior nurses present (Jones, 1968a, pp. 95-8). It was intended that this should become a closed confidential meeting with the focus on interpersonal difficulties, problem-solving and

process. There were distinct problems of transference where the tutor was concerned, and I would have found it much easier to take this group without him. (In retrospect it seems clear that I too had both a transference and territorial problem in relation to this young, predominantly female, group.) However, the nursing staff and the students generally felt this would be un- fair to the tutor, and saw me as trying to devalue him. I agreed to try to work through this with the student nurses as a whole, provided the tutor and I had a review after the meeting itself so that we could learn from one another.

Multiple leadership
Problems of leadership were still given a great deal of attention. For instance, at the twelve o'clock research seminar started by Joy Tuxford, David Anderson (the head social worker) said he wanted to discuss his role relationship with Joy who was also a trained social worker. He then gave a very honest and straight- forward account of his feelings, which I recorded in my weekly diary as follows.

> David understood Joy's research role when she was going around interviewing the various family doctors, but now she was concerning herself with hard data, doing statistics, and at the same time becoming increasingly involved in policy- making; and, as he put it, 'doing a lot of my nagging'. He thought that after twenty years working together, Joy and I had become so identified with the therapeutic community that anyone else must feel at a disadvantage and feel almost com- pelled to go along with our ideology. Joy immediately countered this by saying that therapeutic community was not a static thing, and that the ideology was constantly changing accord- ing to the people in it and the circumstances which existed at any one time. David then continued that he felt Joy was a much better social worker than he was and that he needed her help. However, her close relationship with me and the way in which we complemented each other meant that people felt ex- cluded from getting close to either of us. One of the three senior doctors joined in at this point and said he agreed with David. Joy admitted we had a very close understanding, hav- ing worked together for so long, and that we did, of course, gossip quite a bit, but she felt it was always with the good of Dingleton in mind.
> Joy and I frequently disagree and often find disagreements useful learning situations. I reminded David of the time when I had asked if Joy could act as a consultant and help the Berwickshire team in its community functioning. This had been refused by the social work department, an act which I thought was extremely petty. I feel clumsy and inadequate as a com- munity psychiatrist and want all the help I can get. I would have liked to work with David in the community because I am beginning to understand him better and am really quite en-

vious of Dr Lindsay Madew who is the lucky one working with
David.

Staff roles - hospital v. community
David said he had no wish to be a mirror image of myself in the
community with the overall responsibility for community psychiatry analogous to my hospital role. Lindsay said he would not
tolerate David being community-centred to the exclusion of the
needs of the Selkirkshire team and his own particular needs
within the wards. Under the circumstances I could hardly be
blamed for turning to Joy for guidance in community psychiatry,
when her experience and involvement were relatively greater
than anyone else's. David had no one to blame but himself for
the fact that Joy was competing in an area which was really his.
I told David I very much wanted to confront him with his increas
ing involvement in the power structure at Dingleton, and in a
way this was the very thing of which he was accusing Joy.
It seemed we were going to have difficulty in talking about community psychiatry as an entity, just as it was difficult nowadays
to talk about Dingleton as a whole. The county system, and
particularly the team identities, were tending to create three
little Dingletons, both intramurally and extramurally, and unless
we were careful this might well dilute our collective creative
achievement. However, to offset this was the fact that the two
o'clock meeting on Mondays attended by all the doctors and socia
workers was becoming effective for the discussion of feelings,
and it was here that the various differences within the social
work department and the allied disciplines were discussed.
    The rivalries of senior staff just described point to our limited
skill in resolving our interpersonal difficulties despite many
regularly scheduled meetings for this very purpose. Our
problem-solving skills did seem to improve with experience, but
there is always the limiting human factor!

Decentralization: functional v. geographical areas
About the middle of 1967 we began to discuss a more effective
social organization for Dingleton. There were two main courses
open. One was to divide the hospital on a functional basis with
due regard to the type of disability, length of stay, rehabilitatic
prospects, and so on. The alternative was to think in terms of
discrete geographical areas served by the county teams which
were already established as far as the admission wards were
concerned. During the first half of 1967 the hospital had two
admission wards, a male and female, representing about 38 beds
The remainder of the hospital was made up of long-stay and
geriatric wards, with the exception of the mentally retarded war
which had 37 beds for both sexes. We had, however, not been
able to convince ourselves that we should decentralize the entire
hospital into three separate units. Discussions on this topic
occurred at all levels of staff, but patients were not formally
involved at this time because it was felt this would be irrespon-

sible with the longer stay and more confused patients. It was
felt they should be included when we had definite plans to discuss with them. We were concerned with organizing the patient
population into three major subdivisions, each of which would
include many minor subgroups. The major functional categories
at present were as follows. (a) The short-term new admission,
who usually stayed only two to eight weeks in hospital, were
identified mainly with their own admission-ward area and had
relatively less investment in the hospital as a whole, (b) The
long-stay patients included a spectrum from recent admissions
who had not left the hospital within two months of their admission
to patients who had spent twenty, thirty or even forty years in
hospital. (Many of the re-admissions really belonged in this
category, although in the first instance they were treated as a
new admission in the thirty-bed admission ward.) (c) The
geriatric patients were people showing marked evidence of senile
deterioration. (Many of the patients who were over 65 years old
were not in the geriatric wards, but rather were treated in the
long-stay wards.) (d) A fourth category of mentally retarded
patients were housed in Glenkinnon Ward.

Our problem was to decide which was the more important practical type of division. A division of the hospital into clinical/
functional categories involved such possible categories as:
short-stay new admissions; medium-stay admissions and re-
admissions; long-stay patients with reasonable prospects of
being rehabilitated to the outside community; long-stay patients
who must be rehabilitated to the fullest possible life in hospital;
recoverable, mostly functional, senile psychoses; geriatric
patients with mostly organic disorders who were unlikely to
recover; and finally, the relatively small group of mentally retarded.

The alternative to this clinical or functional stratification of
the hospital population was a geographical selection. New admissions would be dealt with on a county basis by the three
county teams: (a) Roxburghshire; (b) Selkirkshire and part of
Peeblesshire; and (c) Berwickshire. If we carried out a programme of complete decentralization it would amount to dividing
the hospital into three minor hospitals, each county dealing with
its own patients of approximately the same number. This would
mean that clinical or functional groups would give way to geographical consideration. The advantages of the latter were
obvious. The link between the hospital and the outside environment of the patient was strengthened, continuity of treatment
by the same staff personnel simplified, the participation by
family doctors and others in the work of the hospital facilitated,
as was the link between the hospital personnel and the treatment
resources in the community.

The disadvantages were that with our limited physical structure, segregation according to clinical and functional classifi-
cation within the county units would necessarily be limited.
Berwickshire, for instance, had only ten recent admissions at

that time and it was unlikely that we could provide a special ward for these ten patients. The same argument applied if the 37 mentally retarded patients in their ward were distributed among three county units. Clearly, compromises were possible, such as the sharing of admission wards, both adult and geriatric so that all three counties came together on these wards. If the geographical pattern was developed, then any transfer from admission wards to the long-stay or long-stay geriatric wards would automatically be done by referral to the county unit. In other words, we could have three county units for the long-stay and geriatric population, but retain the present admission adult and geriatric wards with all three counties together. This would mean that of our total of approximately 400 beds, 74 would be jointly administered by the three county units and the remainder would be administered separately by the three counties in separate geographical areas.

We reached a compromise between the decentralized geographical and the functional models. These changes enhanced the fluid structure envisaged for geriatric patients in the Borders as a whole. The newly formed Geriatric Working Party hoped to abolish the barriers between Sanderson, an assessment unit some miles distant from Dingleton for geriatric physical cases, Dingleton, the chronic sick hospitals and the Eventide Homes run by the local authorities for the mildly incapacitated elderly. The links with the community would, we hoped, become stronger when each county 'adopted' its own Dingleton unit.

On 8 July I went on two weeks' vacation, confidently expecting that the geriatric decentralization into mixed county wards would be completed during my absence. In fact nothing happened at this time, and it was not until the end of the year that the decentralization actually took place. This illustrated how, after weeks of deliberation involving most hospital personnel, action did not follow. I am not sure why this was, but can only suggest that although we felt we were ready, there was not sufficient motivation to effect the change at that time. Linked with this may be the fact that the patients were not directly involved in the planning. It also suggests that despite our ideal of multiple leadership being largely realized, my role as overall hospital leader tended to linger on.

EXTRAMURAL DEVELOPMENTS

Hospital and Community Services Co-ordinating Committees
The year 1967 saw a great deal of activity in the community organizational field. The Consultative Committee for the Co-ordination of Mental Health Services in the Borders had been meeting quarterly since September 1965. This body had representation from the local authorities of Berwickshire, Peeblesshire, Roxburghshire and Selkirkshire, as well as two general practitioners and representatives from the hospital service.

There was an obvious need for a combined organization covering everyone in the field of general medicine. A Health Co-ordinating Committee came into being at the end of January 1967. At their quarterly meeting in December 1966 the Mental Health Service Consultative Committee had raised the need for a Geriatric Working Party, but it was not until 4 July 1967 that a Geriatric Sub-committee met, under the auspices of both the Mental Health Services Consultative Committee and the Committee for the Co-ordination of Health Services. The joint working party had a membership comprising a representative from the general practitioners; the superintendent of the two hospitals, Dingleton and Peel, who represented the hospital service; a Medical Officer of Health; a welfare officer who represented the local authority service; a psychiatric social worker who had a joint appointment with both Dingleton and the local authority service. The committee met on eight occasions, including four open meetings which were attended by an average of thirty field workers from various hospitals for the chronic sick and the local authority Eventide Homes. In February 1969 a report was published. The following recommendations were made:

1. There is an urgent need for the appointment of a Consultant Geriatrician to act as co-ordinator of the total resources in the Border counties.
2. From the proposed current Register of the Elderly [prepared by local authorities in relation to areas] general practitioners and nurses should maintain contact on a regular basis with their patients in order to anticipate, whenever possible, emergencies or crisis situations. The advisory service offered by the geriatrician's team of field workers should be available as required to all three present arms of the service [hospitals, family doctors and local authorities].
3. Out-patient clinics should be set up in selected areas on a regular basis to be made widely known to general practitioners.
4. The base for the consultant geriatrician with in-patient beds and the necessary ancillary services should be at Dingleton Hospital.
5. The provision of Day Centres at Galashiels and Hawick should be arranged as an experiment with extensions in due course to other viable centres of population.
6. Community care, as opposed to in-patient hospital care, should be critically analysed and valued.
7. A review of local authority allocations and obligations is necessary in order to provide increased medical aids in the home. This is to include physiotherapy and other allied treatment aids.
8. The administrative and communication system should be reviewed so that as much complete information as possible is made available to planners, especially architects, when

housing schemes or residential homes are under consideration.

9. Voluntary agencies should be given much more encouragement and support to provide additional accommodation and schemes for the care of the elderly.

10. We have endeavoured to identify some of the problems; there are no doubt others. We hope our recommendations will be used as a means toward providing in future an adequate and more efficient service.

11. The implementation of the recommendations will mean many consultations and discussions with all major interests; but we believe that the administrative structure in future should be such that all those concerned with the care of the elderly can make positive contributions toward the formulation of policy.

12. It is recommended that a small permanent Advisory Committee, representative of all interests, should continue and be available for consultation whenever necessary.

Borders Health and Social Service Consultative Committee
In September 1967 the two committees covering the fields of mental health and general medicine were joined to form the Borders Health and Social Service Consultative Committee. The following account of its function and continuing evolution was recorded in my weekly diary.

The Borders Health and Social Service Consultative Committee now meets every three months. The original chairman was the county clerk of Roxburghshire; and the secretary is Jimmy Millar, the secretary and treasurer of Dingleton Hospital. This committee has no executive power, but through its representatives conveys the views of the committee to their various employing bodies. The committee has as its major goal the integration of health services in the Border counties. For me it has proved a frustrating but, at times, exciting body. Dr Brotherston, the Chief Medical Officer for Scotland and an imaginative planner, sees this committee as a highly important development and hopes that we will establish a model integrated health service which can be studied and modified for use in other parts of Scotland. The Border counties are a relatively small, compact unit of population involving only 100,000 people. It is possible to know fairly well all the members of the committee, and there are unusually good opportunities for informal discussion and planning. Working with this committee I have learned a great deal about the difficulty inherent in bringing together people from widely different fields in the health service even though they are all striving toward a single goal of improved health facilities.

Factors contributing to this difficulty in interpretation include the family doctors who view the local authority personnel with circumspection. Within the local authority itself there

seems to be relatively little communication or even understanding among the county clerks, the Medical Officers of Health
and the welfare officers. Public health (district) nurses who
are under the jurisdiction of the local authority, but whose
work brings them into daily contact with the family doctors,
hold a highly important but rather anomalous position between
the two bodies. One measure of the growth in the effectiveness
of the committee's work is the trend toward a closer relationship between district nurses and family doctors, and ultimately
a formal attachment to specific general practitioners. The 68
family doctors practising in the Borders have their local
medical committees, but seem to have relatively little influence
in effecting change in their circumstances as doctors. They
seem to be much less firmly embedded in the National Health
Service than either the Peel General Hospital or Dingleton. I
am impressed by the immense support we get from our own
Board of Management, and in a more remote sense, from the
Regional Board. In other words, the three arms of the health
service - hospitals, family doctors and local authorities - have
vastly different terms of reference, and inevitably any one
problem has to be viewed from the differing perspectives of
those concerned. The representatives of these three arms of
the service, meeting in committee, have considerable difficulty
in understanding one another, but regular meetings help to
improve communication and understanding.

By the end of 1967 I had had two years' association with these
various committees and had begun to appreciate how slow-moving
local authorities must be. The officials had to deal with lay
committees who tended to view with disfavour any expenditure
which might increase the cost to the taxpayer. The members of
the local authority were not usually professionally trained people
and were relatively ignorant on matters pertaining to medicine
and psychiatry. I hoped I would be asked to join the appropriate
medical committee of at least one of these authorities, but this
never occurred. Any suggestion of change in the direction of a
more integrated health programme had first of all to pass through
the appropriate committees of each of the four county local
authorities. Integration into one health service threatened the
independence of each of the four separate local authorities. I
started off by believing rather idealistically and, as I later
learned, unrealistically, that the people who live in the Borders,
no matter what their vocation, would be able to unite under one
single identity.
I knew from my experience at Dingleton that rapid change
within a psychiatric hospital could occur, and that considerable
support could be expected from the Regional Board who were
part of the National Health Service. I slowly realized that this
was vastly different from the machinery operating in the local
authority where the terms of reference were quite different and
the outlook of people in power was largely conditioned by the

political and economic aspects of local government. Apart altogether from the social organization, the opportunity for using
learning as a social process with a view to change was vastly
different in the local authority system compared to the Dingleton
Hospital system. At Dingleton the whole emphasis was on social
organization, analysis of behaviour, examining what we were
doing and why we were doing it. Such a social structure made it
possible to bring about change with relative ease. There was no
comparable organization to enhance learning in the other bodies
associated with our co-ordinating committees. The local authorities, the general hospital and the family doctors had little or no
investment in a flexible social organization geared to change.
As a result, although at committee meetings it was possible to
understand the agenda and discussion in a strictly factual way,
the problems of leadership, decision-making, hidden agendas,
and so on were unfamiliar to the vast majority of the committee.

Absence of citizen involvement
At this stage of our development we had paid relatively little
attention to bringing about change through contact with the
citizens outside the formal structure of the local authority and
medicine. However, some awareness of this need began to
appear and we showed interest in the application of therapeutic
community principles in the outside community. We were offered
a house in Galashiels as a possible hostel for our ex-patients
and a party went to inspect the premises. We were very conscious of the interest we aroused in the people living in the
neighbouring houses, and became involved in conversation with
them. We saw that it would be possible to build on this embryonic
communication network, and have some of the local householders
organize some form of committee or supervisory body which
could give local support to the hostel personnel.
  Communication and rumour seemed to have an inverse relationship. By initially involving the local population with us we
avoided the possibility of a crisis developing through misunderstanding followed by confrontation. We saw it as desirable to
apply the concept of prevention so that no misunderstanding or
crisis could develop. The Border Forum which we had helped to
initiate in 1965 was an attempt to bring about some change in
public attitudes by using the appeal of some of the acknowledged
leaders within Borders' society, and by providing a forum where
problems of living could be discussed. We started with highly
topical problems which were bound to interest a considerable
number of people living in the area: the threatened closure of
the railway, the plans for development of industry in the Borders
and the educational system attracted fairly good audiences and
quite lively discussion. However, when we tried to get into
areas where citizen participation and increased responsibility
was called for, we met little response. Particularly disappointing
were meetings held on successive weeks in Galashiels and Hawick,
the two largest towns in our area. On both occasions we dis-

cussed the problem of the aged and how the local community could help the needy older person to remain at home, or at least in the community without having to be institutionalized. At the Galashiels meeting we had an attendance of approximately eighty, 50 per cent of whom must have come from Dingleton. The discussion was quite good, but the absence of a single doctor or minister from the locality was disappointing.

In February the meeting of the Border Forum concerned itself with the relationship between young and adults. We had a turn-out of about a hundred people in Galashiels, and the panel consisted of senior pupils from the local school with Michael Clark, our Principal Nursing Officer, acting as the liaison between the panel and the audience who sat in circles around the panel. The young people apparently had no expectation that what they said would be well received or even interesting to the adults. The Rector from the local school spoke very reasonably, and indicated he was quite willing to allow senior pupils to have regularly scheduled contact with the interested public.

It had already been arranged that I would talk with some of his senior pupils in the near future. I met the sixth form two weeks later in the presence of the Rector. We talked about many things, including psychodelic drugs. The pupils showed interest but lack of information about these drugs. They seemed willing to accept the fact that people turned to them in much the way that some did to alcohol as an escape from painful reality; or in the case of the young, as a new experience. They decided for themselves that turning to drugs increased rather than lessened any problems they might have, and seemed convinced that using drugs solved nothing. There was a lot of talk locally about psychodelic drugs at that time, and I was rung up by two newspapers and by a television service to get my views. I took a very anti-sensationalist line, deploring the tendency to arouse emotional interest as opposed to factual knowledge about this whole problem.

Psychiatric social work
During 1967 our own psychiatric social work department developed in an unobtrusive and unexciting way. At the beginning of the year the Medical Officer of Health for Peeblesshire made some pointed criticism of our social work department, saying they had made little or no use of his own personnel in the field, and obviously devalued our psychiatric social workers. After the meeting I managed to arrange for the Medical Officer of Health and some of his department to meet myself and two of our social workers. In this meeting it emerged that David Anderson, our head social worker, had in fact made little or no effort to involve the Peeblesshire Welfare Office. David explained this on the ground that his first priority was to form relationships with the Peeblesshire family doctors, and felt he could best do this on his own. This led to a discussion of the resistance which most general practitioners showed toward local authority officials,

associating them with the bad old days of duly authorized
officers and the poorhouse. The Medical Officer of Health was
very fair, and an extraordinary situation emerged in which he
finally perceived us as the best sponsors for the role of the
local authority personnel in the community health field. He saw
we were more likely to increase the confidence general practitioners had in local authorities, if we sponsored their cause
and worked closely with them.

It seemed there were three major choices for the social workers.
First to limit their role to after-care, which meant essentially
following up patients who had been in hospital, or dealing with
patients referred as out-patients. The second choice was to have
an extended extramural role and link up much more with the
family doctors, mental welfare officers and the district nurses
in the community. Or third, to emphasize continuity of care
which would mean getting involved in the patient admission
evaluation sessions at Dingleton and helping to make a social
prescription at that time. This seemed to be a much more sophisticated and valuable role to play, particularly if combined with
the second option. We were still a long way from integrating the
social services.

The Monday meeting with the social workers concerned itself
primarily with feelings around the role of the social worker in
the community. Iris Short, the social worker we shared with the
local authority, was leaving at the end of the month (August
1967) and we discussed the qualities which her successor
would need to have. In describing her role, primarily in relation
to the family doctor, Iris said she saw herself, first as a com-
municator, mainly feeding back details about patients who had
been referred to Dingleton; then, as someone to give emotional
support and to educate, primarily by explaining Dingleton to
the family doctor and the ways in which we might be able to
offer help; and finally, as a consultant when the family doctors
sought direct help in relation to a patient whom Iris might or
might not have seen. She felt that something similar happened
in relation to the local authority welfare officers, and she had
set up regular visits with them, which amounted to discussing
areas of mutual help and problems in general. Iris also met the
district nurses regularly, as well as the public health doctors,
and discussed with them problems of administration, policy, role
relationships, and so on. She was asked how far the role which
she had carved out for herself represented the projection of
her own personality, and how far it was a professional social
work role. She felt it was a bit of both. She had made no mention
of the word 'treatment', nor had she mentioned out-patient
treatment or prevention. I asked how often people were being
referred to her by the family doctors with a view to prevention.
She felt the team were becoming comfortable with the Roxburgh
general practitioners and that both she and Dr Todd, the head
of the Dingleton Roxburgh team, were being told about people
who caused the general practitioners anxiety, but who might

not necessarily have psychiatric symptoms. In other words, it
seemed that by not using the 'impressive' approach of the mental
health consultant, and by being a very ordinary person, a social
worker in her role was more likely to pick up the anxieties of the
general practitioners in an informal way, and thus get on to
early cases. At the same time, some family doctors seemed to
prefer to approach the psychiatrist formally as a consultant.

It was generally agreed that the county team should be
approachable through any of its members, psychiatrist, social
worker or nurse, so that the outside community was in a position
to use them in the way that was most comfortable for them. The
general feeling was that we were succeeding in becoming
accepted, and the family doctors were comfortable enough to
talk about ordinary problems of everyday life. They no longer
feared the risk of being talked down to by the psychiatrist, or
being laughed at for making an irrelevant referral or seeing
psychiatric cases where none existed.

Links with the university
By the end of 1967 we began to get some sign of growing interest
from the University of Edinburgh. The Professor of Social Work,
the Professor of Social Medicine and the Professor of Psychiatry
all expressed an interest in using our facilities for training and
teaching. Professor Morris Carstairs, head of the Department
of Psychiatry, had been a great support all along, and indeed
had been partly responsible for my coming to Dingleton in the
first place. The Department of Social Medicine was responsible
for training Medical Officers of Health. As in other countries,
public health was no longer primarily concerned with epidemi-
ology, but was becoming increasingly concerned with the wider
aspects of health and mental health. The Professor of Social
Medicine indicated that he wanted to rationalize the whole question of medical treatment so that it was geared to the actual
needs of the community as they appeared in epidemiological
surveys. There was also the need to train administrators to
operate in regional boards and in the new area health boards
which were anticipated as part of a new integrated health service
in Scotland. Dingleton was seen as a valuable training resource
because of our hospital organization and our attempt to organize
community health services for the counties which we served. Joy
Tuxford's research into community attitudes to mental health was
also of great interest to all three departments.

These overtures from the university departments were more
than welcome and did a great deal to boost our morale. At the
same time, we were fully aware of the embryonic state of our
knowledge in relation to community psychiatry and all that it
seemed to imply. We were far from convinced that the psychiatrist had any significant role to play in the community. We also
felt very critical of the training a psychiatrist receives, which
seemed to us to be quite inappropriate as a preparation for work
in the community.

SUMMARY OF THE FIFTH YEAR

This year saw a further move in the decentralization process. We
spent many hours discussing the relative merits of geographical
versus functional units, and eventually agreed on a compromise.
The three county teams would continue to share the admission
ward and a geriatric assessment unit. The special unit for
mentally retarded would continue as before, shared by all three
teams; but the remainder of the hospital wards, approximately
75 per cent of the patient population, would be run by the
counties themselves.

The physical structure of the hospital made possible such a
move and allowed relatives of patients, family doctors and others
to have some proprietary interest in a ward which 'belonged'
to their county.

Nothing succeeds like success, and our growing reputation as
a good place to work, learn and grow was reflected in our
recruitment figures. Thus, we had only seven nurses in training
five years ago, and now we had fifty. Training opportunities
ranged from a short two-year training for pupil nurses, to three
years for student nurses, a one-year post-graduate course, and
a one-year advanced course in collaboration with the University
of Edinburgh.

But along with this apparent success was a realization that our
enthusiasm might be blinding us to our limitations. We put most
of our emphasis on group work, which included large group
meetings of patients and staff which were usually daily and
brought us nearer to the patients' world; and small psychotherapy groups with selected patients, for example adolescents
and family groups. Staff members all attended training groups,
on the basis that if staff could not resolve their own interpersonal conflicts on a team, then they were not ready to 'treat'
patients! In fact we came to see little difference between treatment and training, and used the terms interchangeably. Linked
to this was our growing interest in what I later came to call the
social ecology of the hospital. This included a preoccupation
with the social structure of the entire system, the roles and
role relationships of staff, patients, relatives and significant
others in the outside world - family doctors, ministers, employers, etc. The physical environment was also high on our list
of priorities. Added to this were the therapeutic community
principles of two-way communication of thoughts and feelings,
listening, interacting, identification of problems, setting of
priorities and social learning. It is easy to see how we tended to
devalue the traditional techniques of treatment, individual psychotherapy, pharmacotherapy and various forms of physical
treatment like electro convulsive therapy (ECT.) But we tried to
add these traditional therapies to our primary social psychiatry
orientation when appropriate. At that time no one believed that
social psychiatry as we practised it was a specific treatment
modality, but that it was an essential component of an effective

treatment programme largely neglected by psychiatry in general. We saw ourselves as a pilot project in this field and lived to see our philosophy given lip service at least in most, if not all, psychiatric facilities in the UK, USA and in Europe.

The final form of the three county teams emerged at the end of 1967, and almost inevitably the major thrust switched from the hospital to the development of effective community services with each county team developing its own model.

Co-ordination of services intramurally, mainly through the SSC, helped to maintain a hospital identity and avoided splitting into three separate discordant county units. But co-ordination of services extramurally was another matter as each agency had its own priorities and territoriality took precedence over a pooling of interests to effect the maximum good for the consumer. However, the Co-ordinating Committee for the Borders continued to meet and we launched a Geriatric Working Party which started in July 1967 and issued its final report in February 1969.

A further development was the fusion of the Consultative Committee for the Co-ordination of Mental Health Services for the Borders, which we had started in September 1965, with its counterpart in general medicine, sponsored by the local general hospital. In September 1967 the Borders Health and Social Service Consultative Committee came into being for the purpose of co-ordinating all health services for the Borders.

Our infiltration into the community continued rapidly, thanks to the three county-community teams and their growing links with the family doctors and local authority personnel in their areas. The two-year-old Border Forum continued to meet periodically in public halls to discuss problems associated with health education.

Chapter 6

The sixth year, 1968:
pending centralization of the health services
in Scotland leads to fear of bureaucratization

INTRODUCTION

The sixth year began with a feeling of optimism. We enjoyed
very positive support from the three university departments in
Edinburgh, and Dr Brotherston, the Chief Medical Officer for
Scotland, gave us increasingly active support and encouragement. Several times he visited us during the year and recognized
the significance of our pilot project as an example of an integrated
health service for the Borders. He was largely responsible for
the Green Paper, *Administrative Reorganization of the Scottish
Health Services,* issued by the Scottish Home and Health Department (1968) and which epitomized on a national scale what we
were trying to do in a minor way in the Borders.

The laissez-faire Conservative government of 1951-64 had been
replaced by a Labour government with an active social policy.
The Social Work (Scotland) Act of 1968 established three separate
departments: Health and Welfare; Children; and Probation.
These were later integrated into one service run by the various
regional local authority social work departments. Thus, social
work was eventually split off from the health services. All this
pending change in the caring services in Scotland looked like
progressive legislation, but with hindsight I doubt if many
people realized the negative aspects of bureaucratization which
followed. My own reaction was to question the wisdom of separating social work from the health services as our own experience
at Dingleton showed that the complementarity of the two services
was beneficial to both. Our psychiatric practice could never
have penetrated as effectively into the community we served
without our social work department. And without them our growing integration with the family doctors, the local authorities,
etc., would have been almost impossible to achieve. In a similar
way social work lost its medical orientation and training benefits
which accrued from close contact with the various disciplines
associated with a comprehensive psychiatric service. All this
impending change produced a drastic effect on our plans for an
integrated health service in the Borders.

For me, the year concluded with a feeling of some disillusionment because of the slow evolution toward such an integration.
I think I was unrealistically enthusiastic and felt that local authorities and medical bodies could change rapidly by internal informal rearrangements rather than wait for pending legislation. I
believed, rightly or wrongly, that if a first-rate co-ordinated

service had come into being in the Borders and had proved its
worth, then legislators would be loath to interfere with such a
structure. I did not, I think, pay sufficient attention to the lay
committees which had the power in local government and were
understandably concerned about the taxpayer's money. The real
trouble lay in the fact that in addition to the plan outlined in
the Green Paper (Scottish Home and Health Department, 1968),
the Social Work (Scotland) Act had been published, which indicated that social work organizations were to exist as a separate
service outside the health service, and as part of the local
authority system. However, the Wheatley Report was not yet
published, and the four counties associated with the Borders
understandably preferred to wait for the findings of this commission. If, as seemed probable, the Borders were to form one
of the local authority regions, then the social work departments
associated with each of the four counties would have to integrate.
I had hoped this sort of integration could take place unofficially
without waiting for instructions from Edinburgh. However, in
fairness, it must be said this was probably asking too much of
people whose future seemed so full of uncertainty. The situation
was made even more complex by the fact that the reorganization
of the health services would bring about a regionalization involving much larger areas than the present areas for which regional
boards were responsible. The new area health boards proposed
in the Green Paper would, we hoped, coincide with the local
authority revised boundaries. The reorganization and integration
of health services could take many years, but my argument all
along was that a successful pilot scheme run in the Borders
would be invaluable as a model for change, and in this we were
given every encouragement by Dr Brotherston to experiment.

INTRAMURAL DEVELOPMENTS

Leadership
The year started with an effective multiple leadership at Dingleton represented by the various disciplines; I had experienced
the difficulties associated with only one authority figure (myself
as superintendent) and was greatly relieved by this development.
It was possible to have an uninvolved leader in any situation
where the formal leadership was threatened and emotionally involved. The whole process of social learning, it seemed, was
greatly enhanced when multiple leadership was a reality, and the
resulting flexibility contributed to a high morale and willingness
to change.

In the spring of 1968 several of the six multiple leaders left,
and I found myself forced into a more active leadership role. The
insecurity ensuing the loss of trusted leaders resulted in my
being put in what I called a 'headmaster' role. I was expected to
give more positive direction than when we enjoyed multiple leadership and was, of course, available to act as scapegoat if things

went wrong! I felt I was not adequately supported when I was in difficulty, and was relatively vulnerable because frequently there was not an uninvolved alternate leader to analyse crisis situations, particularly those in which I was involved. My dual role of physician superintendent and leader of the Berwickshire team became increasingly arduous, and finally, when I returned from a trip to the USA in May, I was informed that I was no longer the team leader. Fair enough! My poor attendance at the Berwickshire team meetings deserved replacement by a very competent nurse. Later in the year my role was further confused by the fact that the three county units which had been launched in October 1966 were beginning to operate independently of hospital policy, resulting in an obscured hospital identity. This, I felt, was partly attributable to my inadequacy and discomfort with regressing to the primary leader for the whole hospital. Nevertheless, the daily meetings of the Senior Staff Committee assured hospital-wide communication and the practice of shared decision-making continued to operate.

In October, following an absence in the USA and Canada, I came back to discover further changes. I had protested my 'headmaster' role and the relative disappearance of multiple leadership, but knew it would take time for new leaders to emerge. Partly to hasten this process the Senior Staff Committee felt I should be less ubiquitous and a member of fewer training groups. In the past I had been an active participant in practically every sensitivity training group. This was a splendid way of gaining an overall view of what was happening at a feeling level within the hospital. It was felt that if I vacated this ubiquitous role it would underline the need for new leaders to appear, and with this I entirely agreed. It did mean, however, that the SSC now had to assume the responsibility for the hospital as a whole, juggling the hospital's interests with the team interests which were at variance. At the end of the year Joy Tuxford, a very powerful leader, made it known that in the autumn of 1969 she was leaving to work in the USA. Although not finally resolved, it became apparent that I, too, might be going to the USA about the same time. During this period Joy Tuxford became a 'bad object', much criticized, and was the brunt of displaced anger emanating from my potential departure, as well as the anger aroused by her own exit.

From the year's outset Joy Tuxford, David Anderson and I met weekly to discuss the possibility of writing a book on our community programme and its development. As the year developed these meetings were viewed by others as possessing some sinister character, excluding the other senior staff, and implying that we were planning the future of Dingleton on a unilateral basis. Interestingly enough, it was only about this time that David Anderson had begun to accept a more forceful leadership role. It was not until October, almost three years after his arrival at Dingleton, that he felt ready as a leader identified with therapeutic community principles to assume an active and

aggressive role in the community. This he did with great sensitivity and skill. But I think it is important to recognize that
such a competent person felt a long apprenticeship was necessary
in a therapeutic community setting before he felt able and confident to apply such principles, modified according to circumstance
in the community. This experience of David Anderson's in relation to an active leadership role highlights the whole problem
of leadership in a therapeutic community - it is a long and painful process when contrary to one's upbringing. People with
formal responsibility, such as consultant psychiatrists, heads
of social work, nursing or other departments, the hospital secretary, and so on, although carrying a great deal of responsibility and power, might never become creative and active leaders
in the psychodynamic and developmental sense. They might make
a relatively small contribution to the process of change or of
social learning, but are able to be effective in their own area of
competence.

What became increasingly clear during 1968 was that the
several leaders whose disappearance meant such a severe loss
were people who had been prepared to get involved in group
process both emotionally and intellectually. The crucial factor
appeared to be their willingness to be available and open to
scrutiny of their performance. In this way they represented a
significant factor in the whole process of learning and change.
Without this type of involvement an authority figure tended to
remain static, and in a comparatively short time this tended to
be seen as passive conformity, within an ever-changing social
organization.

The Hospital Secretary was in a conflicting position. Serving
the Hospital Board of Management and through them, the
Regional Board, their expectations of his performance were pre-
dictability, reliability and conformity to the mores of the
department. On the other hand, as a member of the SSC, he
was constantly influenced by the changing culture at Dingleton.
As secretary to the Dingleton Board of Management he was frequently aware of the absurdities of a bureaucratic machine, with
its lack of shared decision-making, limitations in two-way communication and the difficulties in effecting change. Jimmy Millar
played this dual function with immense skill and courage; but
for him, the whole development at Dingleton would have been of
a much more limited kind! Moreover, his daily exposure to the
largely medical problems discussed and decided at the SSC gave
him a sensitivity to clinical work which administrators rarely
have. The reverse was equally true - as clinicians we became
appreciative of his difficulties in the administrative world.

Other authority figures had to choose between conformity and
risking a negative image within their own professional group.
Michael Clark, the Principal Nursing Officer, was faced by the
need to 'join the establishment' of British nursing if he was to be
seen by them as a competent and reliable administrator. It
seemed to me that the pressure to conform was equally strong in

both the medical and nursing professions. At the same time we were aware that experimentation with new roles and new practice was mandatory if we were to progress. In brief, leadership of the kind we tried to develop in a therapeutic community implied a willingness and a desire to deviate in order to test out new ideas. But it also demanded a sensitivity and respect for the mores of society and the opinions of others, a sense of timing, a willingness to have one's performance scrutinized, and a belief in the value of consensus which really signified trust in the system. Given these prerequisites and a practical demonstration of these qualities, it became apparent that any member of the staff was a potential leader, and by implication a facilitating teacher.

Care of the aged in the community and in the hospital
The Geriatric Subcommittee initiated in July 1967 had done an excellent job in highlighting problems of old people living in the Borders. A nurse was seconded to act as a liaison between the local authority Eventide Homes and Dingleton. We appointed a full-time general practitioner to look after the physical health of our elderly patients in hospital. And decentralization into three county units fostered the senior psychiatrists' awareness and understanding of the problems of their own particular county - specifically, the plight of the aged. As a consequence of our altered admission policy, most requests for admission from family doctors were met by a home visit. The male/female geriatric ward associated with each county enjoyed a strong appeal and positive image which linked Dingleton and the personnel concerned with the care of the aged in the community.

An expanding interest in the geriatric wards was apparent. The new emphasis was demonstrated by several factors. There was, in the first instance, a heightened awareness that old people need not hurry to get up in the morning; allowed to dress as leisurely and independently as possible, they benefit from quite an amount of exercise, and problems of toiletting, etc., are spread over a much longer period. There was improved communication between night and day staff. A less rigid bedtime system was introduced. The tendency to get people to bed as soon as possible to lessen the work for the night staff coming on duty has little to do with the well-being of old people; old people should go to bed when they are tired, resulting in a diminution of the amount of sedative needed. A nap after lunch is physiologically sensible, and makes for a much more balanced day. The daytime activities were associated with familiar aspects of their past daily lives, for instance, baking, cleaning shoes, knitting, mending clothes, and so on.

The change in morale in the geriatric wards was striking. The weekly seminars with the geriatric ward staff surged with interest in the problems of ageing. We began to wonder how far the culture of the geriatric wards reflected our own ideas and fears about dying rather than the actual feelings of people as

they approached death. There was an awareness that we needed
to visit other psychiatric hospitals and study their geriatric
practices. One of the staff had been to St Christopher's Hospice
in London, where there is a special interest in the process of
dying. Probably most important of all was the fact that the
charge nurses experienced a new lease of life, partly because
of increased training and partly because they began to feel
their job in the geriatric and long-stay wards was valued. A
research project carried out by an outside agency helped to
reinforce our impressions, and through their excellent report
stimulated a great deal of valuable discussion.

Work therapy and activity therapy
In conjunction with the decentralization of the geriatric wards,
both in development and in time, we reorganized the work
therapy and activity therapy programmes, basing them with the
teams rather than centrally. We hoped the teams would employ
these activity programmes in a way that augmented their own
perception of the role of the geriatric patient. This attempted
integration of the activity therapy personnel into the teams, and
particularly with the nursing staff, was not altogether successful. Only one county, Roxburghshire, made significant use of
the potential within this scheme. By the end of the year we
realized that the numerous demands on the county teams pre-
vented their giving the activity programmes the kind of attention
in the geriatric wards which was required. In order to properly
attend to their special problems, it was felt that recentralization
of the work therapy and activity therapy programmes was
necessary.
  We decided to separate the work therapy and activity therapy
departments more sharply than in the past. Work therapy would
concern itself primarily with the admission wards, the rehabilitation ward and the ward for mentally retarded patients. The
largest long-stay ward and the four geriatric wards would be
the special concern of the activity therapists. Work therapy
provided supervision in the form of a full-time worker in the
laundry, dining halls, kitchen, the home group (cleaning), the
canteen and the patient assistant nurse (PAN) programme. The
activity therapy programme was staffed by seven young activity
assistants between the ages of 16 and $17\frac{1}{2}$ years old, and a varying number of volunteers who were usually in their late teens
and awaiting university entrance. These young people interacted
with the elderly patients in a delightfully spontaneous way.
There was no set routine and they were encouraged to use their
initiative. Activities included walks, reading to the blind, community singing, card and other games, music, and music-and-
movement (simple exercises and games to music), helping with
meals, bedtime, etc. Their supervisor was a young college
graduate and they had their own training and sensitivity groups.
  One of the APNOs and myself ensured that problems of the
work and activity therapists were given a high priority in the

hospital as a whole. This centralized programme proved to be
much more effective than the decentralized team programme,
because it seemed a minority group like the activity therapists
needed to have its own identity. For this they needed their own
discussion groups with support from experienced and innovative
people. Through this process they had the opportunity to
develop a specific theory and practice, freed from the domination
of a more limiting and authoritarian team-and-ward structure.

EXTRAMURAL DEVELOPMENTS

While waiting for the emergence of several strong leaders so that
our ideal of multiple leadership in a multidisciplinary setting
could be re-established, concern about leadership in the community was growing. For a balanced programme it seemed to many
of us that not only must we have multiple leadership within
Dingleton, but that a parallel development was needed in the
community. However, before such an ideal could even be considered with any clarity, a strong leader within the community
was felt necessary.

David Anderson had joined the staff at Dingleton in the spring
of 1965. By October 1968 David, after three years of relative
ineffectiveness, proved to be an extraordinarily useful leader
of the social workers, and of the county teams generally in the
community. He started by trying to establish effective links
with each of the 68 family doctors through regularly scheduled
meetings. The form these meetings took depended largely on the
preference of the doctor or of the group practice. The keynote
was to allow the family doctors to establish a role relationship
of a kind which made them feel comfortable. This might be at
the cottage hospital with other doctors practising in that area,
or by some arrangement with the doctor alone. Frequently the
most comfortable contact was over discussion of a patient causing the doctor anxiety, but this was not necessarily so.

The family doctors were encouraged to express their views
about the hospital team practice and to indicate how they preferred to interact with the team: either with the psychiatrist,
the social worker, the nurse or through a combination of these.
Once a comfortable relationship was established, it was much
easier to discuss possible variations of roles and role relationships with a view to improving effective functioning. As a by-
product of this active exploratory role in the community, the
Wednesday afternoon community services meeting which most
of the staff attended, with Joy Tuxford acting as facilitator,
became of extraordinary interest. Each of the three teams spent
twenty minutes describing exactly how they were interacting
with the family doctors and in general defining and refining
their community roles. Having spent most of my professional
life in hospitals, I was in a situation similar to most of my colleagues in having to learn a new role appropriate for extramural

work. Joy, by contrast, had had many years of exposure to
social problems in the outside environment. She had done the
original follow-up study at Henderson in the early 1950s (Tuxford, 1952), and at that time taught me most of what I knew
about outside social agencies concerning welfare, probation,
rehabilitation, etc.

By playing a peripatetic role and, in collaboration with Joy,
reinforcing the work of the social workers and the teams
generally, David became an invaluable teacher doing what
amounted to an action-research job. David's leadership in the
extramural dimension also implied a satisfactory role relationship
with the various social agencies in the community. However,
difficulties are inevitable in an integration of differing disciplines
in the health field in the outside community.

Social workers seek identity outside the National Health Service
By November 1968 we heard rumours that the Royal Commission
on Local Authority Reorganisation (Wheatley Report) might
recommend that the south of Scotland be divided into either one
or two regions and that our social work direction might well come
from some remote central body. My reaction to this rumour was
noted in my weekly journal:

> The opportunity for social work and health to be closely inte-
> grated in one department is past unless something quite un-
> expected happens. Jimmy Millar, the Hospital Secretary, has
> been talking with the county clerk who was engaged in draft-
> ing a proposal for his new social welfare programme which
> would be for Roxburghshire alone. The other two Borders
> counties refused to come in, so that instead of one social work
> service we are going to be faced probably by three separate
> services, which makes no sense at all. I began to feel that all
> our work in bringing about the Borders Health and Social
> Services Co-ordinating Committee was going to be wasted, and
> felt we ought to call an emergency meeting of this committee
> to discuss our failure to achieve an integrated health service
> for the Borders. On Monday at the Administrative Meeting I
> suggested this emergency meeting of the Co-ordinating Com-
> mittee, and Jimmy Millar said he would get in touch with the
> county clerk, the chairman of the Co-ordinating Committee,
> and try to arrange such a meeting. At the SSC I tried to
> continue this discussion, but when I talked about the tragedy
> of social work developing its own unified service at the ex-
> pense of health as a totality, the chairman, David Anderson,
> told me to shut up! I respected the chair, but reserved the
> right to continue discussing this matter at the two o'clock
> social work meeting. At twelve o'clock at the Berwickshire
> team meeting, Jill, a nurse, and David fed back that they got
> the impression from the local authority officials whom they had
> just met at Duns that Berwickshire was probably going to with-
> draw from our joint-user scheme, and pay their own part-time

social worker. At lunch I talked with Jimmy Millar and raised
the necessity of working out an arrangement whereby Jill, a
nurse acting as a social worker, could be upgraded from her
status and pay of staff nurse to that of a full member of the
social work department, paid at about the level of a charge
nurse. This would mean, of course, that she would no longer
be seconded from the nursing staff but would be a fully paid
member of the social work department. Jimmy thought this
might be done.

It is interesting to note that a year later Berwickshire
appointed a community nurse to work with the Berwickshire
county team. Betty Stobie did an outstanding job in developing
this new role as described in a paper written in collaboration
with the team psychiatrist (Stobie and Hopkins, 1972).

At the two o'clock social work meeting David, as chairman,
allowed topics to be raised which seemed to me to be avoiding
the main issue. I got angry, saying that far and away the most
important matter for the whole meeting was to consider calling
an emergency meeting of the Borders Health and Social Service
Co-ordinating Committee. This was discussed with considerable
feeling, and David wanted to know why I was so anxious. I
pointed out that we still had the trump card to play if we
could get Dr Brotherston to back the Borders as a special
case where a pilot project, based on health integrated with the
social services, could be carried out. All the evidence pointed
in the opposite direction, and unless something desperate was
done we would simply find ourselves being ruled by some
central authority and with a bipartite instead of an integrated
service. Joy and David both lessened the tension of the meeting immediately before the end by very sensible comments
regarding what lay behind the tension. It seemed that David,
as a social worker, was reconciled to the need for social work
on a national scale to establish its own identity, and Joy
pointed out that I had been acting as a doctor and, by suggesting that nurses could become social workers, was anticipating
the possibility of medicine having to 'go it alone' if the relationships with social work became too strained, and the local
authority and hospital services became separated.
   At 5.00 p.m. when Joy, David and I met as usual, we inevitably discussed the events of the day, and all agreed that it
had been a very constructive, although painful, experience.
In a way we had all been angry with the situation which was
emerging and about which we could do little or nothing. I was
angry with social work in general for being so stupid, at the
same time sympathizing with David and his department at
Dingleton which might well be destroyed by the more highly
paid local authority social work programmes. I was preparing
to meet this threat by seeing nurses being trained to become
social workers, so that Dingleton would not be without a source

of recruitment. It became clear that our only course was to
obtain sanction to have a social work department which was
outside Whitley Council (National Health Service) scales of
pay and was competitive with the local authority system. If
this could be done we had little doubt that social workers
working in an integrated team at Dingleton were far better
off than social workers who were working more or less in
isolation under the local authority. Our experience when visiting some of the best examples of local authority programmes
in the UK suggested that it was very dull when social workers
operated together in isolation and not as part of a multidisciplinary team. We realized that some of our present
troubles might have been less had we had the foresight to
make contact with the leaders in the community. Thus, David,
who had been recommended by both Joy and myself to get
close to the county clerks, had failed to do so. Moreover,
David might well have been offered the position of leader of
the new social work department which each of the local authorities must plan. [He was, in fact, later approached on the
subject.] Finally, we were hoping to put the Co-ordinating
Committee to the test to see if it was just a lot of talk or if it
really had courage and power. If they could not agree about
such an integrated service among themselves, then we could
not expect Dr Brotherston to have any belief in us as a
Borders community.

Opposition from the Borders Health and Social Consultative Committee

In December 1968 came another severe disappointment when the
Borders Quarterly Co-ordinating Committee for Mental and
Social Services met. The chairman and county clerk for Roxburghshire set the tone for a most negative attitude on the
part of the local authorities. They apparently felt unwilling
to take any active steps in an integrated health service for the
Borders in view of the imminence of the Wheatley Report, which
was a Royal Commission on local authorities to be published in a
few months' time. I got quite angry and said the whole point of
our committee was to bring about integration in anticipation of
legislation rather than waiting for it! The latter course meant
that we would simply be told what to do from Edinburgh, and I
believed that if we developed a well-integrated service before
the advent of legislation, no one would be very keen to destroy
it. This independent approach met with some response from the
doctors present, but only blocking from the local authority personnel. The most we could do was to set up an ad-hoc committee
to look into the working of the Social Work (Scotland) Act with
a view to having at least a unified social work service for the
Borders which would include Dingleton. I was pointedly left out
of this committee, although, in fairness to the chairman, I
received a rather apologetic letter from him afterwards. I said
that future generations in the Borders would have little to thank

our committee for, and that legislation would inevitably be
suited for large urban communities rather than for a rural one
like the Borders. A ray of hope came later when we had a letter
from Dr Brotherston saying he was sorry that he had not been
able to be present at the meeting himself, and suggested that Mr
Millar and I might like to meet him and Professor Morrison, head
of the Social Medicine Department, in Edinburgh. The fact remained, however, that far from feeling excited about the possibility of bringing about change quickly in the Borders, I became
resigned to the fact that this would take longer than I thought
– an example which, for me, was painful communication and
learning. Jimmy Millar, however, remained a beacon of hope and
nothing would dim his enthusiasm and belief in the future of the
Borders.

Should I leave Dingleton?
By the end of the year I was still pretty content with my lot,
but at the same time felt the need for a change. I started work
at Dingleton almost exactly six years ago and was beginning to
find that certain aspects of the role of superintendent were
repetitive. Doctors and individuals from other disciplines came
and went, and with few exceptions left just when they were
becoming useful. The core staff of people, like David and Reg
and some of the new nurses, gave one a feeling of accomplish-
ment and reward. Administrative people like Jimmy Millar and
my secretary, Cathy Wilson, were unique, and I will never
know their like again. However, when one considered the
temporary staff, the 'chronic' nurses and others, my role had
become less satisfying. I was growing a little tired of these
repetitive situations, and was showing my impatience by acting
more unilaterally than was consistent with the hospital culture.
    There were other factors contributing to my restlessness. The
railway line closed on 6 January, which made nonsense of the
Borders Development Plan, which hoped to bring new industries
into the Borders. This plan itself had been held up because a
landowner refused to give up his land, and in the light of these
developments, any new industry was very doubtful about the
wisdom of coming to the south of Scotland. There was also much
quarrelling among the various townships regarding their participation in any development plan. We dropped the Border Forum
largely due to a lack of community response, which was sympto-
matic of the feeling that some of us had that no strong Borders
identity existed, or at least we had failed to mobilize one.

SUMMARY OF THE SIXTH YEAR

The impending reorganization of the health services in Scotland
with new legislation affecting hospitals and their community
services, a social work service in process of being divorced
from the National Health Service and absorbed by the local

authorities, and a reorganized local authority system whose
boundaries might or might not coincide with the new area health
boards all caused an atmosphere of uncertainty in the Borders
and elsewhere in Scotland.

I knew that our six years of work at Dingleton, which had
accomplished the nucleus of an effective integrated mental health
service for the Borders, was seen by Dr Brotherston, the Chief
Medical Officer for Scotland, as a valuable pilot project. We even
entertained the idea that if we had a viable community health
programme in reality, we might influence the planners to leave
us alone to continue our project. Grandiose thinking maybe, but
when Dr Brotherston's Green Paper, a health plan for Scotland,
finally appeared it bore many similarities to our own work
(Scottish Home and Health Department, 1968). My fear was that
a small rural area like the Borders would inevitably have to sub-
mit to plans designed for the vastly more populous urban areas
of Scotland, and that the new area health boards would include
populations far in excess of our 100,000 people, with all the
attendant problems of a remote invisible bureaucracy.

However, our aspirations proved to be unrealistic, and the
Borders authorities on the Borders Health and Social Service
Consultative Committee, with whom we had to work, were in no
mood for heroics or risk-taking. Understandably, the three
county local authorities were preoccupied with their own individual fates, particularly as the Wheatley Report on Local Authority Reorganisation had not yet been published. The family
doctors were supportive but lacked money, a strong organization
or an effective parliamentary lobby.

As we learned later (after my departure), our worst fears
regarding the bureaucratization of area health boards and local
authority social services were realized! And we had the doubtful
comfort of knowing that what we achieved in forming, in part
at least - an integrated mental health system in the south of
Scotland - would have been nearly impossible after the new area
health boards went into operation. The freedom and intimacy of
our own Board of Management for Dingleton was to disappear to
be replaced by a faceless bureaucracy run by people who are
often too far removed from the patient world to have any hope of
knowing or understanding the very people whom they purport to
serve.

This disillusionment in the community field did not negatively
affect our intra-hospital evolution, partly because Jimmy Millar
and myself were the only people directly involved at the socio-
political level as committee members, and partly because the
hospital was to some extent self-contained and had plenty of
internal problems to occupy it fully.

As planned, multiple leadership and shared decision-making
inevitably eroded my power; my wish to delegate authority and
responsibility to the system had been a guiding principle from
the start. This transition was dramatically illustrated when,
during my absence in the USA, the Berwickshire team dropped

me as their psychiatrist and team leader, and substituted a competent nurse whose attendance could be depended on! They retained my assistant, Jean Smith, as a psychiatrist.

Another portent of change was an SSC decision to limit my ubiquitous role. I was involved in most of the training seminars and sensitivity training groups throughout the hospital. Following the departure of several of our acknowledged leaders, an attempt was made to lock me into my original superintendent role. This I resisted successfully and helped in the process of re-establishing multiple leadership. But the SSC pointed out quite rationally that this process would be better implemented if I made more room for alternate leaders – I was slowly doing myself out of a job!

The saga of David, the head social worker, is thought-provoking in this context of leadership. For three years he kept a low profile, learning therapeutic community principles and later social work in the community by being a member of one of the three county teams. He stubbornly resisted assuming his formal role of head of the whole department until he understood how to implement therapeutic community principles in the community. When he at last felt competent to be an effective leader, he performed with outstanding success!

Chapter 7

The seventh year, 1969:
a leadership crisis and an exciting liaison
with the local school system

INTRODUCTION

The events of 1969 occurred on a background of my possible departure from Dingleton, and the fluctuating emotions aroused by speculation, anxiety, unrest and anger. My deputy, Dan Jones, showed no eagerness to replace me. Although he had been recruited as Deputy Physician Superintendent two years previously, he had always kept a low profile and was content with his role as leader of the Roxburghshire team, where he was an outstanding success. The rest of the senior staff resisted assuming extended leadership roles, and Jimmy Millar faced a serious crisis as described later. This temporary upset in our established multiple leadership pattern forced me to face a vacuum at the top which was resolved quickly and demonstrates how regression can be one dimension of growth. In response to these circumstances my role changed considerably with more emphasis on training and less on administration. In the community we became much more closely involved with the local high schools, largely due to an empathetic new Director of Education.

INTRAMURAL DEVELOPMENTS

My departure
The onset of the year brought with it a strong suspicion that I would be leaving Dingleton sometime during 1969. My decision was not finalized until I paid my annual consulting visit to the USA in April and accepted an offer to start work in September 1969 at Fort Logan Mental Health Center in Denver, Colorado. My decision was prompted by numerous factors, the most important being my disinclination to face retirement at the age of 65, which would ensue automatically if I remained in the National Health Service. Fort Logan appealed to me in its own right because I had been associated with it since its inception in 1961, and had been privileged to visit as a consultant facilitator every year since. Their approach was very similar to our own and I had developed great respect and liking for the people there. It seemed to me that it was one of the most, if not *the* most, significant state hospital in the USA. A dramatic change from the old hierarchical structured state hospital, it attempted to deal as far as possible with patients on a day-hospital basis and in the community. Therapeutic community principles were practised to an extent

which I had not found elsewhere. Even before I was totally certain of my departure, there was a strong probability that this would happen. Thus, most of 1969 seemed to have been a preparation for leaving.

The resignation of a key person in any institution inevitably arouses a large amount of speculation, unrest, anxiety and anger. We felt that if Dingleton had a flexible social organization and was responsive to the need for change, we should be in a position to circumvent many of the negative aspects of separation

Unsettled state of the senior staff

At the beginning of the year, at the doctor-senior nurse sensitivity training group, we discussed Dan Jones's leadership potential in the event of my leaving. He talked about his fear of assuming a leadership role in a therapeutic community. He had been quite happy as the doctor on a Himalayan mountain-climbing expedition, but found himself less comfortable leading a county team at Dingleton. He thought he would not be able to take over my role at Dingleton if I left. In February the same sensitivity training group addressed itself to the future of Dingleton, assuming, as seemed probable, that Joy Tuxford, Michael Clark and myself would all be leaving sometime in 1969. This meant that two doctors, Dan Jones and Carlos Chan; David Anderson, the head social worker; John Sutherland, Deputy Principal Nursing Officer; and Jimmy Millar would be the most senior people with reasonably long experience at Dingleton. They worked through some of their feelings of despondency and began to cheer up when everyone indicated they had no doubt about the wish to continue developing as a therapeutic community and that the main thing was to ensure that my successor also thought along these lines. Although it was unlikely that the Green Paper would be implemented (Scottish Home and Health Department, 1968), or that the Regional Board would disappear in less than five years, they all expressed concern for Jimmy Millar whose world was changing around him. Concurrently the Social Work (Scotland) Act had thrown the social work department into confusion and no one knew what the future of hospital social work departments would be or if they would survive under a hospital salary schedule as well as under a community setting. Recruitment for social workers became increasingly difficult because of the higher pay offered by the local authorities. We had already established a practice of attracting American social workers, and our recent advertisement had realized over forty applications from the USA, despite much lower salaries in the UK. In view of our experience, an agreement was reached that any successful future candidate would be requested to make a commitment of at least two years. This seemed to be the minimum period when an American could both become acculturated to Scotland and contribute usefully.

A bureaucratic trend appears

In February Jimmy Millar's lack of confidence became apparent –
a consequence of my prospective leaving and of his uncertain
future. Despite careful planning to maintain a social work department of six, and Jimmy's agreement to use money allocated
for a psychologist position, we nevertheless had a crisis over
this issue. Dr Hal Shure, who had come to work with us from
Fort Logan Mental Health Center in Denver, Colorado, innocently
precipitated this by saying that, on principle, he would prefer
a psychologist if one could be recruited. Jimmy used this as an
excuse to withdraw his commitment to use the money for a sixth
social worker. He seemed to become a careful bureaucrat – a
sharp distinction from his usual sparkling and enterprising self!
This same trend was reflected in the Hospital Board Meeting
which went on much later than usual, largely due to Jimmy's
pedantry which seemed strangely unfamiliar. At Thursday's
Senior Staff Committee Reg commented on the new Jimmy who
seemed to be bothering about bureaucratic details in a completely
new way. It was almost as though Jimmy had joined Michael Clark
in becoming a good civil servant.

The uneasiness created by the upcoming loss of leaders is
depicted in my diary notes:

An interesting factor in the situation was the difficulty in
getting David Anderson, the head social worker; John Sutherland, the most senior remaining nurse; or two of the doctors,
Dan Jones and Carlos Chan, to assume leadership roles. They
were the only senior people available to maintain a continuity
of the therapeutic community ideas. I was trying to pull out,
but instead of these four filling the vacuum, there was a
tendency for Dr Shure, a newcomer, to become a leader. This
represented a rather confusing artefact because Dr Shure
made it clear that he will be returning to the USA at the end
of the year. I spoke to Dr Dan Jones, who seemed to see the
danger very clearly, and admitted that he might unconsciously
be manipulating Dr Shure to play this role because of his own
diffidence. As the senior consultant, Dan realizes that no
matter what happens he will be formally responsible for medical
matters, particularly in relation to the outside world. Joy
Tuxford's very useful role was limited because of her own
pending departure. She and Reg seemed to be seeing the situation more clearly than anyone else, but I saw a danger of
their becoming associated with myself and therefore automatically 'bad'. Under the circumstances there was a kind of
leadership vacuum, and almost any enterprising individual
could be sucked in. Clearly the leaders had to declare themselves and endeavour to re-establish contact with Jimmy, if he
was to be given the confidence to resume his previously enterprising and 'marginally delinquent' role in administration.

Change of leadership means re-examination of values
The continuing process of working through leadership issues,
my leadership role as a 'leaving leader', and evaluation of the
values and beliefs held by a system in change - are further
portrayed in my diary notes describing a sensitivity training
group at the end of March (Jones, 1968a, pp. 95-8).

At the sensitivity training group Dr Hal Shure said he felt he
was constantly finding himself in a position of criticizing me,
and Dr Dan Jones said he, too, felt a need to oppose me. Dr
Carlos Chan joined in and made some critical remarks about
my performance. We looked at the whole question of values,
the role I had played in the past, and at the gaps that had
been created by my withdrawing from the various training
groups in preparation for my departure (but mainly as a
result of pressure from the SSC). Hal then questioned if what
I saw as important would be perpetuated in the new value
structure which would emerge after I left. Reg was quoted as
being my protégé along with other nurses like Beryl Hume,
and it was suggested that in the new order, confrontation and
other techniques which I favoured might be devalued. Reg
was criticized as seeing any falling away from the familiar
structure as regressing. There is some truth in this, and it
seemed clear that for the first time people who are staying on
after I leave are beginning to develop their own therapeutic
culture which need not necessarily follow the old pattern. This
seems appropriate to me, provided it does not mean reverting
to the traditional hospital structure, because that means a
more passive, dependent role for patients and staff with less
opportunity for growth. The question of whether I should with
draw completely from patient-staff involvement was discussed,
and differing opinions were expressed. Hal wanted me to remain active, and to learn from me while I am still at Dingleton;
Dan felt he could not operate if I simply step aside and wait
for him to fill a vacuum. He wanted me either to operate fully
or not at all.

A new model for leadership
As Dr Dan Jones, my deputy, had no wish to take my place as
superintendent, I thought we might try to transpose David
Anderson, the head social worker, in my place. However, on
talking with Jimmy Millar, and the chairman and vice-chairman
of the Board of Management, I became convinced this would
arouse too much opposition from the medical profession: we
would be much wiser to try a 'cabal'. This implied that the three
senior doctors, the director of nursing and the senior social
worker would form a policy or steering committee with Jimmy
Millar in attendance to represent the Board of Management. This
group would then be in a position to elect their own chairman
and vice-chairman. If this had turned out to be David, then any
medical matters could be dealt with by a medical vice-chairman

who would deal with the Senior Administrative Medical Officer at
the Regional Board, and so on. This would ensure a democratic
organization with multiple leadership giving equal status to the
Hospital Secretary, doctors, nurses and social workers at least
intramurally. Everyone at Dingleton seemed to like the idea, and
David felt this was much more appropriate than having to deal
with the hostility of the medical profession if he had been appointed superintendent. We knew we would have to raise David's
salary in order to keep him at Dingleton. However, quite independently of this, he had decided not to apply for the
Roxburghshire social work directorship (at twice the salary)
because he felt the frustrations associated with the local authority
would be too much.

My diminishing authority and responsibility
The continued shaping of my role by the system is revealed in
my diary notes recounting a June sensitivity training group
attended by all the doctors and social workers:

> Jan Houston, a social worker from the USA, said how irritated
> she was by my tendency to make them feel guilty and devalue
> their performance. This followed my expressing disappointment
> at their attempt to explain Dingleton to a group of medical
> administrators from the Usher Institute, the Social Medicine
> Department of the University of Edinburgh. Michael Grieve,
> another social worker, disagreed, feeling that I was only being
> consistent with learning theory and painful communication.
> Hal Shure said he was just beginning to grasp the real message
> of Dingleton and how our practice was relevant to social action
> generally. Frank, the new doctor, said he wanted to learn and
> Joy refused to be drawn, preferring a low profile as she her-
> self was leaving. Apart from these individuals, the general
> feeling of the group was that they could not be themselves and
> grow while I was around. The feeling was that I should absent
> myself from everything except the 8.30 a.m. meeting, where I
> could continue in my administrative role, leaving Dan free to
> get on with his clinical role.

I further recorded in my diary, summing up the events of the
week:

> I tried to help this metamorphosis by saying I really wanted to
> leave Dingleton by making a positive contribution, and that the
> more time I had to write up a developmental history of Dingle-
> ton, the better I could do this. Having taken the plunge by
> saying that they want me out of the way, the group seemed to
> reflect an immediate feeling of relief and accomplishment. It
> was as though they had shown how powerful they were and
> how vulnerable even I was! This feeling of elation affects me
> too, because I feel proud of their accomplishment and relieved
> that I am allowed to give them a present in the form of a seven-

year report on the process of change at Dingleton. The situation has a certain reality too, because, thanks to our unusually favourable recruitment, we have enough doctors this summer to make it feasible. [In fact, we had four doctors, for periods of time varying from two months to a year, and one medical student, all unpaid by us and extra to our establishment. This seemed to be a measure of the growing interest in therapeutic communities in Europe and the US.] I realized that the person who would be most affected, Jimmy, was not at the meeting. I asked Joy if she would come with me and see Jimmy and she agreed. Jimmy was most grateful to be informed before this news was fed back to the 8.30 and the SSC. His immediate response was one of sadness and some anger with the other 'silly fellows'. He was warm and appreciative of the support he felt he always had from me, and dreaded the future in case an adequate replacement for me was not forthcoming. However, he was philosophical and accepted that if this was what people wanted and if it was ratified by the SSC, he would go along with it.

After seeing Jimmy I began to feel thoroughly depressed and took a walk through the grounds as a kind of symbolic departure. I met a group of old men patients who greeted me cheerily in the sunshine. I saw Kerstin, my wife, just back from Edinburgh. She waved cheerfully and, in reply to my question; 'What do you think I am feeling?' she said – 'You're in the process of leaving, aren't you?' – which I thought was an astute bit of intuition.

My diary notes continued:

On Wednesday at the 8.30 I tried to get a minute to discuss my departure but failed. It was interesting that when it came to priorities at the SSC, no one mentioned the need to discuss my role in the light of Tuesday's sensitivity training group. I was forced rather ignominiously to ask if I could discuss my own funeral! Interestingly enough, Dan took the lead in discussing what had happened, and gave a fair enough representation of the way in which leadership would emerge more spontaneously if I was not present; and that I had asked to be relieved of official duties so that I might get on with writing up a developmental history of Dingleton during the past seven years.

Hal made it clear that he did not understand the idea expressed, that either one had to be fully involved or not at all. Reg was Reg, saying he was sorry this sort of thing was necessary at all, but supposed that if this was what I wanted, then he would go along with it. Jimmy had to be invited to speak and he also made it clear that he was very upset, but that he would go along with the consensus. Not for the first time, the SSC looked unable to make up its mind, and so I tried to help them by saying I definitely wanted to be left alone

to do some writing. However, probably wisely and as chairman,
David said he felt the SSC was not quite able to take the sudden change in circumstances; and in view of the Glasgow
University Television Team's visit on Thursday and Friday, it
would be better if I would remain in the SSC this week. However, I was assured that I would get a final decision by Friday.
I asked to be allowed to play a teaching role and interact with
visitors, and it was suggested that we might even have a
special seminar once a week to look at the process of change
and use it as a teaching opportunity in addition to my present
regularly scheduled Thursday evening seminars on therapeutic
community principles. On the whole, I felt that the SSC had
done the best job possible under the circumstances, and said
I doubted if my leaving could have happened in such a sophisticated manner in any other institution in the country.

On Thursday the SSC operated under the glare of television
lights; I think it was a fairly typical day that was videotaped,
starting with the 8.30, then the SSC, then a discussion on the
intramural and extramural structure and function of Dingleton.
This videotape is still used for teaching seminars at Dingleton
and gives a graphic picture of the process of change in relation
to my leaving and the staff's skill in working through this
problem. Finally, the usual Thursday night seminar with pupils
and teachers from Roxburghshire, attended by around sixty
people, was videotaped. The videotape of the SSC meeting on
that day should be quite historic. The SSC managed to finalize
their decision to ask me to withdraw from all Dingleton activities other than teaching, in order that I could apply myself to
working on the history of Dingleton. The discussion took much
the turn of the previous day's SSC, and the feeling of transition was heightened by the fact that we had news from Michael
Clark that he had been accepted as the Head Nurse in the
largest group of hospitals in England. I think he is glad to be
going as administration is his major interest and he feels
frustrated by the expectations of a clinical role which the
therapeutic culture demands of all staff no matter how senior.
He has a brilliant mind and has done a splendid job in developing an unusually flexible and able nursing body.

Nursing changes
In the spring of 1969 we had a new intake of nine post-
registration nursing students, three of them from Westminster
Hospital, a London teaching hospital. The calibre of the applicants was excellent! Nursing was booming and the quality of the
applicants steadily rising. It was tragic that Ted Smith, the
Nurse Tutor, was forced by circumstances to resign; he was
not appointed as the Head Tutor of the newly combined nursing
school created by the amalgamation of the nurse training programmes of both Dingleton and Peel, the local general hospital.
It appeared that this trend was apparent all over the country
and that as an integrated training for nurses was approaching,

psychiatry was being pushed into a secondary role by general nursing. What a pity it was to see the UK follow the American pattern, abandoning our separate training programmes for general nursing and psychiatric nursing.

EXTRAMURAL DEVELOPMENTS

Integration with local high schools
In January 1969 we had the first of our meetings with school-teachers from Roxburgh county and Dingleton staff. This was made possible by the new Director of Education, Mr Charles Melville, who shared our interest in the process of learning and felt discussion on this subject would be mutually beneficial to his teachers and Dingleton staff. At the first meeting we discussed the concept of cross-age teaching, which I had learned from Dennie Briggs and it had made a deep impression on me (Lippit and Lohman, 1965). Basically the idea is as follows: A group of children from one particular class who are interested in the possibility of playing a teacher role meet with their teacher for a certain number of meetings to discuss the whole idea of taking on the role of teaching younger children. When they feel sufficiently confident and clear about what is intended, they then each interact with two or three pupils, usually two years their junior. They teach common subjects like maths, reading, history, etc., and after a one-hour teaching session, the older children meet their teacher and discuss their experience. What emerges is a new interest by the older children in the whole idea of teaching, identifying much more with the role of the teacher, and appreciating some of the difficulties that he or she must have. In addition, they begin to wonder about their own prejudice towards younger children, their unwillingness to inter-act with them in the playground, their ideas of superiority, and so on. From this living-learning situation they go on to discuss wider issues to do with prejudice, racial discrimination, and so on. (The idea of cross-age teaching was not new to Scotland; it had developed quite naturally in some of the very small country schools, where a single teacher would utilize her more competent pupils in this way.)

On 20 February I accompanied Mr Charles Melville, the Director of Education for Roxburghshire, to Hawick High School. Two women teachers had implemented what we had discussed at Dingleton at our January meeting, and we saw 14-year-olds teaching 12-year-olds. Mr Melville said he had never seen a class so intent on what they were doing. On talking to the children afterwards, the younger group said they liked equally having a boy or girl teacher, but with the older group it seemed that the boys much preferred to teach boys. It seemed that the older children felt it was a privilege to teach a younger class, and it made them think about the whole meaning of 'teaching'. The younger children said they felt closer to their 'teacher' than to

their real teacher, although they liked the latter. Both the older and younger children talked about their experience with considerable animation, and it apparently opened up quite new perspectives regarding the whole idea of 'school'.

At the end of our afternoon visit to the school we had a tea-time seminar with the teachers who showed a good deal of resistance to two comparative outsiders. They felt threatened that their role was being discussed and that we were having access to 'their' children. However, there was a considerable degree of interest, and we were told that 53 teachers planned to come to the seminar at Dingleton that evening. However, there was heavy snow on the ground and I was astonished to see twenty teachers turn up.

We used a socio-drama technique, creating a problem of stealing at school and asking various members of the staff from both the school and Dingleton to play the various roles. The general feeling among the teachers was that we knew remarkably little about what went on in school; this may have been quite fortunate, as our very ignorance may have helped to stimulate interaction and learning as well as lessening their feelings of vulnerability. The teachers wanted to go on with these seminars, but hoped we could make the subject-matter more specific. Our tendency to let a topic for discussion emerge as a result of informal interaction between those present was new to them. As teachers they wanted to know exactly what we were establishing as our goal for the evening. At this meeting we did stress how impressed we were to think that cross-age teaching, which had been discussed with some of the teachers a month previously and had been brought to their notice for the first time, was actually being practised by two of the teachers at the high school.

In March Charles Melville and I visited Kelso High School. We had lunch in the same room as the pupils, a very noisy experience. We then moved about, dividing up to see different classrooms. I went to Mr Turple, who seemed to be very near to our own ideas about learning as a social process, and I sat in a back desk among the class of fourteen or so boys. This was a class who were not going on to do their O levels and would be leaving school that year. They were addressing themselves to the general problem of 'I'm leavin''. It was really an exercise in communication, and Mr Turple was writing on the blackboard the responses various pupils gave, so there was a sort of build-up which they could all see. They got around to the idea that because they would be leaving school as early drop-outs they were 'different'. I had slipped in quietly and found an empty desk at which to sit and listen. Later I put up my hand and asked what they would think about themselves in a year's time when they were out in jobs, and asked them to compare themselves with their own age-group who stayed in school. They were very fair about this, seeing the advantages and disadvantages pretty clearly. They would have jobs, money, responsibility, more girl-friends and better opportunities for an

early marriage, but this advantage would be lost when the boys who stayed on at school finished and went to the university, etc However, they did feel that in a year's time they would, in fact, be more mature than those who stayed on at school, and we discussed what they meant by the term 'grown-up'. I then asked if one of the boys could take over the class, and Mr Turple willingly sat at one of the desks and let a volunteer take over. This boy did quite well and there was no suggestion of antagonism by the other boys who continued to ask questions and developed the theme very well. It indicated a great deal of role flexibility within this particular group of boys and the security that they felt in Mr Turple's class.

I then met Mr Herriot, a maths teacher, who told me about a fascinating seminar he had had the previous week with about fifteen parents and pupils together. This meeting was arranged in order that parents could understand something about modern mathematics because they could not understand what their children were being taught. This had turned into a useful discussion and it seemed that the parents were surprised how freely and confidently their children spoke in open discussion. Mr Herriot said he had tried this venture because of the stimulus of the last teachers' meeting at Dingleton.

We then saw a few of the 34 very impressive clubs which Kelso High School had developed. Pupils go to these clubs voluntarily provided there are vacancies, but must remain in the same club for a full year. A group of boys were developing plans for the future of Kelso, a town with some 10,000 inhabitants, analysing the accommodation in various hotels, etc., and finding that there were practically no places available for bed and breakfast; also the caravan site was being analysed, playground facilities, and so on. One club was called AAA - Association for Argument and Action - and was led by Mr Turple.

The Rector, Mr Alexander Russell, had been a bit controlling and kept a sharp eye on us during the day from 12.30 onward, but when we reached tea, which was delightfully served in the library at 4.30, we saw a more relaxed picture. Mr Russell allow free discussion at the seminar and we saw the whole spectrum from the rigid person who felt the personality of the teacher was what really mattered, to people like Mr Turple and Mr Herriot, who were clearly willing to see learning as a social process. It was at this meeting that Mr Herriot said that a comment of mine earlier in the day had made him feel ashamed of the fact he was not going to the meeting at Dingleton that evening. He changed his mind and would keep his word to bring along some of his pupils.

The meeting at Dingleton that night had approximately twenty teachers and about the same number of Dingleton staff. Thanks to Mr Herriot's pupils, four boys and one girl, the seminar was quite exciting. The fifth-form pupils took up the challenge from the start and made one realize what a good school Kelso High was. They felt there was a good deal of two-way communication

in all the classes, and even where it was not apparent, the
teacher tended to take the hint from the pupils, and would
interact in response to the pupils' lead. It sounded almost too
good to be true, but when some of the teachers talked about the
same kind of free discussion at university, the meeting split
into two camps: Joy spoke from her past experience at London
School of Economics, Francine (a social worker) from Cape Town
University, and several people from Edinburgh University; all
deplored the rigidity and authoritarian structure which was
characteristic of the social structure of the British university.
I talked of the rigidity of the medical training, and the same
applied to psychology, nursing and so on. A volunteer worker
at Dingleton, who was also a teacher at Galashiels Academy,
helped us to focus and talked about the teaching profession as
she understood it. She emphasized that there was little or no
attempt by the teachers to learn from what they were experienc-
ing with the children, and that there was certainly no structure
for formal seminars or learning theory. The whole meeting was so
absorbingly interesting that 90 minutes had passed like nine!
To me the most striking factor was that the pupils seemed to
have no difficulty in seeing the importance of learning as a
social process, and that it could not be separated from the
acquisition of knowledge with a view to training and passing
exams. They saw teaching and learning as complementary, and
indeed had difficulty in separating the two. It was agreed that
we would invite five pupils to return for the next meeting. It
was also agreed to ask fifth-form pupils from Hawick High School
and from Galashiels Academy to attend, provided the rectors
approved.

It was significant that, for me at least, the most important
aspect of our extramural development at that time was our growing liaison with the schools. During the first half of 1969 we
made a great deal of progress in forming a communication network with some of the schoolteachers and the pupils. Unfortunately, our infiltration in this direction met with much opposition,
and this was understandable and predictable. Nothing had been
achieved previously because we had not the sanctions from
above, nor strong support from within the school system. Ever
since I arrived at Dingleton we had tried to link up with the
schools, and the best we had managed was to have periodic
visits from school-leavers. Although a highly desirable and
modest goal, this was never fully realized. Our hope was that
if every school-leaver in the Borders visited and came to know
something about their local mental hospital, prejudice and misunderstanding, which belonged to the past, would have a chance
of disappearing. Such prejudice was reinforced by parents whose
knowledge of Dingleton was usually very fragmentary, often
based on fantasy, and out of date. We felt the pupils were quite
able, at least in some cases, to educate their parents and bring
them up to date. In a decade all young parents who had grown
up in the Borders would be able to view Dingleton with a much

more informed attitude; this of course would inevitably affect
the attitude of the next generation. Thanks to the support from
the new Director of Education in Roxburghshire, Mr Charles
Melville, we were able to take the process of mutual education
between the schools and Dingleton a stage further. By involving
both teachers *and* students in our joint seminars a situation
developed which had much in common with the problems between
young and old in all 'advanced' countries. Personally I think the
generation gap is a myth which raises false expectations of misunderstanding between young and old. If we expect communication difficulties, we will inevitably find them. My experience
in the last six months had confirmed my belief that it was just
as easy to communicate with young people as with my own age-
group. The crux of the matter was interest and empathy. I
actually developed this theme when I moved to the USA, and
became convinced that there were enormous possibilities for
preventive psychiatry if social learning became as important as
formal subjects taught in schools (Jones and Stanford, 1973;
Jones, 1974).

Social work department
I have said little about our social work department during 1969.
For reasons which I did not fully understand, their activity in
the community seemed to have lessened or at best remained
static. One factor was that David Anderson had been re-
established as a significant leader in the hospital. My pending
departure and withdrawal from an active role created a vacuum
which seemed to draw David back into the leadership struggle.
This was a temporary phenomenon, and he eventually continued
to develop and lead in the extramural dimension. However, this
experience underlined the danger of a hospital service, and
particularly a therapeutic community where the support, interest
and comfort of the hospital was a very powerful force in seduc-
ing individuals to operate from the hospital base rather than in
the community outside.

SUMMARY OF THE SEVENTH YEAR

The process of change during my last year at Dingleton took some
surprising turns. One aspect of this is demonstrated if we follow
the saga of David, the head social worker. In 1968 it looked as
though he had finally reached the goal of leader of the therapeutic
community in the outside community. But with my imminent departure a leadership vacuum appeared. My colleague and deputy,
Dr Dan Jones, indicated clearly that he did not want to take my
place when I finally departed. The only other possible candidate
appeared to be David, but tradition called for a medical superintendent. In fact it appeared that David was not adverse to filling
the leadership vacuum even though he had only recently moved
his focus of interest from the hospital to the outside community.

We had by this time incorporated the principle of multiple leadership in a multidisciplinary setting, but this only applied intramurally. The outside world and the Regional Board in Edinburgh still expected one person, the superintendent, to be answerable for all aspects of the clinical work at Dingleton. By contrast, our own Board of Management were much more sophisticated and accepted the concept that the SSC had a more global view of events than any person alone could have. However, they felt that if David replaced me it would arouse too much opposition from the medical profession. We came to the conclusion that the best course to follow would be to form a 'cabal' involving the three senior doctors, the director of nursing and David. In this way multiple leadership was assured, and Dan Jones could placate the medical profession while still retaining David's leadership skills.

Another anomaly created by my impending departure was the avoidance of overt leadership and risk-taking. Jimmy in particular changed dramatically, became relatively bureaucratic, and to everyone's dismay avoided participation in decision-making or risk-taking, as did the other senior staff members. Dr Hal Shure, a relative newcomer from the USA, became the acting leader by default until the ultimate decision to form a 'cabal' was made.

In line with these developments my remaining hospital authority was significantly reduced, and a modified therapeutic community culture evolved, replacing the familiar one. When, with my connivance, I was ultimately eliminated from the formal social structure of the hospital and left to write my review, everyone, including myself, was relieved.

However, the work of mourning regarding the departures of Michael Clark (the Director of Nursing), Joy and myself was carried out, retrospectively in what was a highly creditable way as described.

The events surrounding changing patterns of leadership during my last year at Dingleton seem to indicate that even when multiple leadership in a multidisciplinary setting has become a reality, there are still certain attributes of authority peculiar to the role of the original leader. Such a conjecture helps to explain the apparent resistance in finding a replacement for me and the difficulty in re-establishing multiple leadership in my absence. This might help to understand Jimmy's reversion to his erstwhile bureaucratic role after seven years of outstanding leadership at Dingleton. Ken Morrice would probably have filled the vacuum had he still been with us, as would David had he been a doctor instead of a social worker - a sad reflection of society's apparent need to trust the medical profession. One additional factor may have been associated with my preference for the role of the facilitator - by helping people to help themselves I may have formed a sort of symbiotic relationship with some people. This would seem to apply to Jimmy in particular. In fact had *he* left Dingleton and I remained, a somewhat similar phenomenon might have happened to me!

Finally, the personal pain of separation was offset by a fascinating experience in social learning through interaction with pupils and staff at the local high schools. Thus, my partial disenchantment with the process of political and bureaucratic change in the community of the Border counties was replaced by a new enthusiasm and task. Preventive psychiatry and social learning in schools seemed to make more sense in the long run than intramural treatment of society's drop-outs in hospital.

I left Dingleton in September 1969 with very mixed feelings. It had been an extremely happy and productive seven years in my work and family life. We had a beautiful home on the hospital grounds, close to Jimmy Millar's home. My three young daughters loved the environment and were a familiar sight in most of the hospital and especially the canteen! The success of an open system in a mental hospital and its surrounds had far exceeded my expectations, and we attracted visitors from all over the world. I was satisfied that our type of therapeutic community represented a treatment methodology in its own right. This belief in our accomplishments and a desire to demonstrate our methods elsewhere, combined with a desire to escape 'retirement', led to my departure for a training post at Fort Logan Mental Health Center in Denver, Colorado.

Chapter 8
Synthesis: what is social learning?

The seven chapters covering my seven years at Dingleton are
based on records written at that time (1962-9). Now, twelve
years later, I am attempting a synthesis of that material, paying
special attention to the concept of social learning and adding
relevant experiences up to the present time.

In the introduction to this book I talked about social learning:
two-way communication motivated by some inner need or stress
leading to the overt or covert expression of feeling and involving cognitive processes and change. The term implies a change
in the individual's attitude and/or beliefs as a result of the
experience. These changes are incorporated and modify his personality and self-image. The fact is that social learning is a
process involving many factors which, according to circumstance,
will have many different combinations and permutations and is
incapable of definition.

The Greek prefix syn- (together with) gives the key to this
chapter. In an attempt to synthesize the concept of social learning I have taken twelve dimensions of social learning from among
many other possible factors and will discuss each one briefly.
But the sum of these twelve dimensions does not add up to social
learning. Nor can social learning be broken down and understood by an analytical process. We have to be circumspect about
the 'scientific' tendency to understand the natural world by
reducing everything to its component parts.

Learning, growth and creativity form part of a continuum in
which the variables interact with each other in relation to some
particular context including the environment. According to
general systems theory nothing can be understood in isolation,
but only as part of a system. And social learning is an ongoing
process which does not stand still, just as our perception of
reality is changing constantly. Social learning cannot be taken
apart and understood by isolating it from its context. The inter-
relationship of the parts is the key. If you separate the parts
the interconnections escape and it is this system of linkage that
is the essence.

When people ask me how I define social learning, I am not
sure what to say or how to respond. It is like asking someone to
define 'love', or 'happiness', or 'beauty'. I think there comes a
time when we must accept that we cannot define, analyse, pull
apart everything in order to understand it. It is almost as if we
do this because we want to 'possess' what we pull apart. We must
also learn to accept the limitations of verbal language and begin

to communicate on other planes and in other ways. Can we explain in words the meaning of an African tribal dance, even if we know the language and culture? Words cannot adequately explain the spiritual, artistic and abstract dimensions. The variables involved in the synthesis would be unique to each individual observer, and would be almost impossible to compare verbally. The temptation in our culture is to verbalize, intellectualize and 'believe' in our conclusion. Our struggle to understand schizophrenia epitomizes this difficulty.

A review of what I learned at Dingleton starts appropriately with a general discussion of social learning. The eleven other factors contributing to the synthesis of social learning are then discussed. No attempt is made to rank these attributes in any order, as each learning situation has its own particular format and all of the factors overlap one another in creating this synthesis called social learning.

SOCIAL LEARNING AND GROWTH

There is nothing new about the concept of social learning. The Socratic method of instruction is 2,000 years old. It is vividly described by Roszak (1978):

> Socrates described himself as a midwife of self-knowledge. The image presents the paradox of a constructive permissiveness. The midwife is one who comes to make a 'delivery', yet she comes empty-handed because what she has to deliver is already there, somebody else's creation and possession. Thus, Socrates does not come to tell the young what to think or how to live. If they ask for such direction, he stymies them; he purports to know nothing. He will only say, 'Let us talk it over'. And he adds, '*You* begin'. As it turns out, his 'ignorance' is a fertile vacuum; it draws out the student's inner resources - tentative ideas, unformed tastes, embryonic aspirations. What the student offers in the dialogue does not always meet with benign indulgence (that would be the course of a treacherous permissiveness). More often it is astutely, but lovingly, criticized. But these *are* authentically the student's own convictions that are being used as experimental raw material. The student opens the dialogue and is encouraged to try out this position and that. Each argument, even if it is angry and abusive, is taken up seriously and examined, until the student sees its limitations or folly. In the course of things, Socrates even criticizes his own convictions and invites the students to join in.

One way to demonstrate social learning in a psychiatric hospital is to have a review immediately following a daily ward meeting involving all patients and staff on a ward. Discussion of the problems of living and human relationships in the ward meeting

are witnessed by everyone, but viewed differently by each individual according to many variables, including personality, educational background, motivation, etc. To turn this shared experience into a learning situation (training) for the staff, a review supervised by a competent facilitator has enormous potential for social learning.

A review is an attempt to 'relive' the process with the staff immediately following the community meeting and examine the group process from beginning to end. Did the group start on time? Who sat beside whom? Did staff form clusters? Who spoke first? And so on. Verbal and nonverbal communication are recycled with a view to examining staff performance. Did we miss a cue, for example an interaction which lent itself to interpretation? Were we defensive, blocking client criticism of our behaviour, or our apparent lack of concern, or our lack of consistency in fulfilling an obligation to honour an agreement made in a previous group, or an apparent 'leak' of confidential material to a higher authority? And so on.

More subtle and demanding is our willingness to listen to criticism from our own peers and to see this criticism as part of a process of social learning and not as a 'put down'. An outside facilitator who is chosen by the staff for his or her group dynamic and social system skills can add significantly to the willingness of staff to listen and learn from their peers. The facilitator has a degree of objectivity which helps to avoid staff splitting into subgroups, etc. He or she can also help as a role model in demonstrating the use of confrontation as a technique for social learning.

A review of this sort that is held daily is a very effective training device. The various personalities and training backgrounds of staff offer differing perspectives and reactions to the same client-staff group. The day in, day out examination of performance may be painful at times, but social learning is often a painful process. To examine in retrospect what one did and why one did it in group interactions heightens everyone's sensitivity and skill. Not only can one focus on such things as the timing, sensitivity and aptness of one's inputs, but the complementarity of staff group members in reinforcing another's inputs can be discussed. For instance, a well-timed interpretation of some defensive client behaviour, for example, the client's unwillingness to talk about a problem of stealing, may result in an opening up of an issue, and if this is handled sensitively by the staff as a whole, the trust level rises and more sharing of potentially threatening issues may ensue.

Some people like to hold a review of this kind in the presence of the clients as silent listeners. With a fairly experienced group this can further enhance the level of trust between clients and staff, and can help blur the distinction between treatment and training.

To apply social learning in a school presents many difficulties. In a school setting the teacher or lecturer usually communicates

information by a one-way process to a captive audience. The subject-matter or curriculum is decided by some distant body of 'specialist' educators who decide 'what is good for' the class. The class interest and involvement has never been tapped and the teacher also may be bored and learn nothing new himself. The social ecology of the classroom is inappropriate for social learning. The seating arrangement in geometrical rows, the confining desks, the teacher's podium and the sterile environment are all conducive to lack of interest. A diversion such as a crisis, for example a fainting attack affecting a student, can immediately invoke interest and an opportunity for social learning. The back-to-back seating is replaced by a curious circle. The teacher may demonstrate his awareness of physiology and psychology of non-reinforcement of anxiety by his studied unconcern and deference to the laws of gravity by leaving the student in his prone position. The natural regrouping and interest in the event may be capitalized by the teacher suggesting that the class sit in a circle and then leading a discussion after an appropriate interval, in which the mechanism of fainting and the virtues of non-intervention are shared.

In brief, this is a plea for as much attention being given to social learning as to teaching (the acquisition of knowledge mainly for later school exams). In most schools the latter predominates and a unique opportunity for growth is lost. Some teachers have a natural aptitude for an open system approach, but in general, extensive training is called for. But where can this be obtained? It is not something for which teacher-training courses are known.

My own experience in this area has been described elsewhere (Jones and Stanford, 1973; Jones, 1974), and involves volunteer teachers in their own training group. After at least three months with a competent facilitator participating in two-hour group-interaction periods per week, the teachers are ready to start informal interaction with their pupils. The facilitator (usually a mental health professional) helps the teacher to gain the pupil's confidence in talking about events in the classroom, playground and outside. It may take months to achieve a level of trust, where personal problems can be shared with the group. Learning to understand what lies behind much of our behaviour, particularly at times of stress, is an experience that seldom occurs in the classroom. The general attitude of society is that the function of school is to impart knowledge necessary to pass exams and as a prelude to being 'qualified' for the job market. Problem-solving and an opportunity to acquire attitudes, values and beliefs to ensure a satisfying and fulfilling life are left largely to chance or assumed to be the responsibility of parents. The emphasis placed by society on conformity further blocks the emergence of an individual's latent creativity and growth. This education in conformity begins, if not in the family itself, certainly in a big way once the child goes to school. Our educational systems stress completing courses and obtaining degrees rather

than developing divergent imaginative thinkers. Most educational settings are characterized by convergent question-asking in which 'the' one correct answer is known by the teacher and is to be memorized by the students to regurgitate for exams. This may be good training for the work world which the student eventually enters. Here the same hierarchy of values exists, and one works for money instead of grades (or marks) as a reward (a healthier system of rewards or of giving value to what one does could be worked out); the only problem is that the problems of school become a bit more difficult to ignore when they become problems of industry; manifested in rising absenteeism, alcoholism, mental illness, declining productivity and quality of work, high rates of divorce, teenage delinquency, etc. - all side-effects of a dysfunctional society in which people often have little involvement or participation. And so our society's problems might well be looked at in relation to the types of social systems in which children are exposed and grow.

From what has been said the reader will realize that no sharp distinction is being made between the fields of mental health and education. Social learning, in my opinion, is as relevant to the school or industry as it is to the mental hospital or other psychiatric facilities. Applied throughout the entire school programme it would represent a significant contribution to preventive medicine and the art of living generally. The full realization of every individual's potential for creativity in a group setting would seem to represent an essential aspect of growth.

Social learning does not imply insight (although this may happen) as in psychoanalytic theory and practice, when the client's unconscious material is made available to his conscious mind. In fact the learning process may not be conceptualized at the time, or be available for instant recall. Rather it may be an 'awareness' - a response from some sensory stimulus communicated through any of our senses and needing some later event before it crystallizes out in one's conscious awareness. But I have observed on many occasions how a change in my own, or someone else's, attitudes, values or beliefs can happen without full awareness at the time of the process involved. If a group of highly motivated students interact in relation to a common problem, it seems reasonable to postulate that no one individual can 'stand still' when listening to his peer's reactions to the problem. His original position (concept, prejudice, uncertainty, etc.) is inevitably modified to some degree. It may produce a change in attitude to the problem which he can articulate, or some subtle change may have occurred outside his awareness (to surface with or without an awareness of the process at some later date). Alternatively, a change may have occurred in his attitude, values or beliefs which he is not aware of until the change is pointed out to him by another person.

I find it difficult to separate the concepts of social learning and growth; they form part of a continuum. George Land has

written extensively on the biology of growth and the correlations
with human development. He says (1973, p. 135):

> In all 'learning' situations, the goal directiveness of organisms
> is the pervasive influence and motivation. If information is not
> perceived as connecting with existing patterns and is not
> viewed as contributing to effect and growth, learning will
> simply not occur. If, on the other hand, any information is
> presented so that it links with existing data and leads to
> growth effects, learning is automatic.

Growth is a natural propensity of all living cells, but is largely
circumvented in man through fear of the unknown and of potential danger to the status quo. Thus, despite endless opportunities
for growth offered to man, relatively few will be accepted.
Growth is a natural phenomenon of all living things, whereas
learning has to do with knowledge acquired from a teacher or
through study, instruction and experience. It is predominantly
an attribute of man and social learning requires social interaction
between people in an appropriate environment.
    Learning as a social process is linked to the concept of a
strong group identity. This is particularly important when the
project entails leaving conformist standards and becoming
'deviant' in the eyes of society.
    The fact that at Dingleton I headed an organization with a
highly integrated culture was a factor in our feeling of invul-
nerability - however illusionary. A group identity is well known
for its value in crisis, for example destroyer crews in wartime
usually had a higher morale than the great battleships, where
a group identity was much less evident.
    This factor of size is enormously important and it is commonly
held that the vast power of the huge corporations will in time
lead to their downfall, and thus to much smaller or decentralized, mainly autonomous units. But even hospitals as small as
Dingleton with only 400 beds have a need to decentralize into
manageable-sized subunits. This happened with the emergence of
the three county units. They were semi-autonomous with their
own social structure and leaders, but remained identified with
the hospital as a whole through daily representation by their
leaders at the daily Senior Staff Committee meetings. Thus, all
personnel had three group identities: (a) hospital, (b) county
and (c) professional discipline, in that order. Even in their
community function, the county community teams retained these
same three identities.
    This holistic model meant that cross-fertilization was con-
stantly occurring as was a stimulating rivalry with the other two
counties. This hospital decentralization has been discussed in
Chapter 4, and the comment was made there that despite all our
efforts to retain a hospital identity, there was a strong temptation to identify with the smaller and more intimate county units.
This highlights the problem in much larger institutions, where

decentralization is inevitably associated with a loss of identity with the parent body.

I believe that all the principles associated with social learning described in this book apply to any social system with appropriate modifications. It would be absurd to apply them literally in an operating theatre at the time when surgery was in progress, but a democratically conducted discussion at the end of the operating session would lead to some surprising revelations for the surgeon regarding not only his behaviour during surgery, but the needs of his junior staff. I have said repeatedly that, given motivation on the part of each individual, interaction, listening and learning follow automatically - it is the 'given' items that are the imponderable factor!

However, social action usually stops short of the initiation of a change process. The need to control, basically a symptom of insecurity, asserts itself as in the case of arbitration. Arbitration aims at an agreement between the two sides involved and, although some social learning may occur, the primary goal is to settle the dispute - an example of when the goal gets in the way of process. Here lies the impracticability, as some people would call it, of the approach recommended in this book. It goes against the authority structure which predominates in the present-day culture. Even if a counterculture of a more democratic kind emerges, as is in fact happening (as described in the final chapter), there would still remain the need for a special training without which social learning cannot effectively function. This is the essential message of this book and implies a long-term plan, starting in elementary school where the principles and practice of social learning can be practised and ultimately become part of our culture.

LEADERSHIP

I was lucky to be associated with a hospital that wanted to change in the direction of an open system; I had been hired with this in mind. My senior colleague, Dr Ken Morrice, had already prepared the way by outlining the possibilities of this approach to some of the senior staff before I even arrived at Dingleton.

I knew, nevertheless, that I was initially imposing *my* ideas on the staff and lost no time in starting the process of shared decision-making and thus aspiring to a group identity. The Senior Staff Committee commenced two days after my arrival, at first meeting twice weekly and later daily. Thus, from the outset, senior staff, representing all areas of hospital functioning, were involved. My innovative role rapidly changed to that of 'one of several' important persons in the shared decision-making process. This occurred gradually, after I had outlined the meaning of an open system as applied to Dingleton. Everyone appeared willing to accept this approach as our long-term

goal, which I emphasized might take years to realize even
partially.

I have often wondered about the use and abuse of my authority
in relation to my role as the leader of a therapeutic community.
At Dingleton I had the formal power as Physician Superintendent,
but liked to claim that this power was never invoked. It was a
latent authority which existed as a last resort in an emergency,
but to which I never resorted. To have done so would have been
folly and the direct antithesis of an open system.

One important aspect of an effective leader in an open system
is his capacity to facilitate learning and growth. Through this
process multiple leadership evolves and the formal leader becomes
primarily a facilitator. Further discussion of the role of the facilitator is continued later in this chapter.

The attributes a leader wishes to demonstrate in the evolving
system would include group as opposed to unilateral decision-
making, risk-taking, focusing on learning, giving positive feedback and criticism, flexibility and openness, resiliency, welcoming
the unexpected, and showing confidence and trust in people - all
essential in sanctioning change.

I felt that one of my functions as the formal leader was to set
the tone for creativity which developed from a supportive but
energetic and enthusiastic experimental attitude. Dogma I avoided
like the plague (or tried to); criticism was welcomed even when
painful. I readily admitted my mistakes, and tried to demonstrate
my own capacity to learn and change. The importance of a role
model as a factor in creative development is discussed further in
Chapter 9.

The climate was that of a supportive group and was almost
always light-hearted rather than serious. If people were going
around glum, cranky and frowning, it was a good cue that much
was amiss! My belief is that the distinction commonly made between work and play is a sad reflection of a limited system. If
people are not enjoying their work, then creativity is limited if
not squelched altogether. Part of our task was to set free the
'child' in the system.

SHARED DECISION-MAKING

I firmly believed that to make a unilateral decision within the
therapeutic community social structure was a mistake, as discussion and interaction with my peers or with the patients
usually led to social learning; and that my original position must
inevitably be modified by listening to other points of view. If no
one chooses to believe me when I say that I never made a unilateral administrative decision, it seems to reflect in part their
unwillingness to adopt a group identity. That a group decision
must, in general, have more validity than an individual one is a
position I can defend on the basis of my experience, but the idea
seems to enrage some people who see this as anything from arro-

gance to dishonesty. It is not a position that can be proved or disproved and, like therapeutic community principles in general, represents a paradigm which suffices as a methodology until further knowledge is available to form a new model.

In the early days at Dingleton we resorted occasionally to voting in order to achieve a rapid decision on some important issues. Even if preceded by discussion involving all parties concerned, there is still the danger of splitting the 'winners' and 'losers' into two factions and thus reinforcing the negative attitudes of the losers. This negates the significance of a decision which ideally has the support of everyone concerned and therefore the motivation to succeed is strong.

CONSENSUS

Consensus implies that every member of the group, irrespective of status, has an opportunity to share his/her views, while at the same time listening to those of the others in the group. The fact that everyone can be heard and his/her point of view considered helps to weld the decision-making process into something approaching uniformity. Nevertheless, the process implies that no one person can get his/her way, and that what emerges is a form of compromise which is seen by the group as being the most viable outcome possible under the circumstances, and worth trying out at least for a trial period.

Decision-making by consensus seems to me to be a common-sense procedure. Why offer oneself as the scapegoat for a social organization when things go wrong? Let everyone relevant be part of the decision-making process and thus be identified with the outcome. Even when this represents failure, the motivation or commitment is there to study the reasons for the failure, and thus learn from it. Incidentally, there is no difficulty in getting everyone to enjoy success and even learn from it!

Consensus decision-making is time-consuming and like all aspects of social learning may be painful, but in my opinion, is mandatory where important decisions are concerned. I think a distinction can be made between shared decision-making and consensus. The former has not the same quality of working through a problem to reach a decision. In consensus everyone is identified with the composite solution agreed to, which involves a considerable amount of time, trust and commitment; and the often painful process of social learning. Shared decision-making is usually less time-consuming and means that, although everyone has some understanding of the different aspects of a problem, no unanimity is achieved; thus, not the same motivation to succeed with the plan adopted as in the case with consensus. Consensus is often used loosely to mean the former, and a useful distinctive quality is lost.

FACILITATOR

An important factor in the avoidance of abuse of power by any
leader is the concept of a facilitator. The facilitator has been
mentioned many times in this book in connection with social
learning (Jones, 1976b), and has an important part to play in
the process of confrontation (Jones, 1976a, pp. 27-38). (Refer
also to Chapter 3.) The term implies that the facilitator plays
the difficult role of holding up a mirror so that the person or
persons involved can be helped to see things as they appear
to others. The facilitator must have the experience and skill to
be trusted by all persons involved and the empathy to encourage the expression of feelings - only then will he/she be listened
to by the people concerned, and social learning proceed.

In a crisis situation involving two or more angry groups, a
more formalized procedure is often called for (Jones and Polak,
1968). The confrontation should occur as soon as possible after
the event, when feelings are high and ego defences relatively
absent. The first necessity is to find someone whom all people
concerned can agree to as the most appropriate facilitator. This
person must be readily available, which implies a flexible social
organization where priorities can be changed quickly - as in the
case described earlier (see p. 73), when I left a Board of
Management meeting at a moment's notice to respond to a request
to facilitate a crisis in the admission ward. With an angry conflict the facilitator needs the authority and skill to restore order
to the extent that people can listen to each other and be exposed
to the opposing view of the conflict. My experience is that social
learning almost invariably follows - whereas to wait for 'tomorrow'
would mean that defences like rationalization and projection had
been formed overnight, and unproductive argument, without
social learning, might result.

This may sound like a veiled authority figure who uses his
power to restore order. But when two disturbed angry factions
have to agree on a facilitator, one faction might hope that the
facilitator will support them and punish their opponents, but
such a person would probably not be chosen by the other group.
To reach agreement regarding an appropriate facilitator, the
choice was usually a mild person whose character was strong but
fair. Here the difference between authoritative and authoritarian
is important. David Anderson was a good example of such a person who frightened no one and had a warm but authoritative
personality.

MULTIPLE LEADERSHIP

The idea of shared decision-making or consensus implies group
rather than individual leadership. I have already discussed my
refusal to make unilateral decisions on the grounds that a group
decision is more balanced and effective than one that I would

make alone. Authority figures frequently make a show of en-
couraging shared decision-making, but ultimately decide for
themselves as though the group was not to be totally trusted.
Such a façade has its uses in terms of information-sharing and
probably has some effect on the decision. But the ideal of multiple leadership in a multidisciplinary setting implies that all
staff have their individual areas of competence, and when these
are recognized should lead to that individual being the leader
in appropriate situations, for example a nurse might be a ward
team leader with a doctor accepting her authority because she
is closer to the ward life.

My first two years at Dingleton were characterized by a difficult leadership situation due largely to the absence of several
alternate leaders. Ken Morrice, as my deputy, was a strong
and reliable assistant, but circumstances and his own good
sense cast him in the role of my main critic - an essential
counterbalance to my sometimes over-enthusiastic and hurried
style. This difficulty contributed to splitting of the staff into
two factions and came to a head after eighteen months. This
was resolved only when two strong personalities, Paul Polak
from the USA and Shail Kumar from India, arrived and were able
to function as alternate leaders. Now if Ken and I were in conflict, one of the two other doctors was able to act as a facilitator,
and so the difficulty was usually resolved and social learning
occurred. It is worth noting that neither Matron nor her deputy,
although they were authority figures, had the group work or
psychodynamic skills to function as facilitators. During my last
three years at Dingleton we had usually six alternate leaders
who could play a facilitator role in the staff meetings, and this
contributed to a remarkable degree of stability in our social
organization. Ultimately, multiple leadership involved people of
all disciplines, and leadership was related more to personality
and skills than to seniority and pay.

CONTAINMENT

I learned after years of painful controversy with my peers that
my own desire for power and control virtually demanded several
strong alternate leaders, any one of whom could act as facilitator
when I was emotionally involved in what often amounted to a
rivalry situation. In other words, although I firmly believed in
a democratic structure and shared decision-making, my natural
tendency was for an active and at times aggressive role which
contradicted my open system beliefs and demanded that I be
'contained'.

This concept of 'containment' applies to any strong leader who
requires equally strong alternate leaders to 'hold up a mirror'
so that he becomes aware of his performance as seen by others.
I both delighted in and hated this aspect of our therapeutic community culture. Without this procedure my own learning and

growth, as well as that of the system, would have been jeopard-
ized. The positive personality attributes are retained; the negative, contained.

SYSTEM SURVIVAL

There is a common misconception that a social organization like
a therapeutic community tends to die with the disappearance of
its original leader. Such an argument overlooks the fact that the
organization, in our case associated with an evolutionary process
covering seven years, had moved from the conceptual paradigm
of the originator, and passed through endless transitions where
the group increasingly took precedence over any one leader. A
therapeutic culture, once established, has the flexibility to
absorb new leaders who add their personality attributes and
beliefs to the system and so change it, but they, for their part,
have to accommodate to the prevailing culture. My experience at
the original therapeutic community in London was that an open
system, once established, is too rewarding to the people in it to
tolerate any newcomer who threatens this individual freedom and
group identity. Henderson Hospital, now 34 years old, is still
an open system. Many things have changed, but not this essential quality. The same general argument applies to Dingleton,
which I left twelve years ago. The formal leaders today, Dr
Stuart Whiteley and Dr Dan Jones, respectively, identify themselves with the same basic principles, and this applies in general
to the staff and patients at these two hospitals.
    An open system of the kind described here continues to grow
and change, and this very vitality is the best safeguard against
institutionalization, a disease process which even sociologists
seem to believe is the inevitable fate of any innovative programme.
Stuart Whiteley, Bob Hinshelwood and Nick Manning have all
worked in open systems and have now increasingly involved other
similar organizations, so that networks are recognized in Scandinavia, Holland, the USA, Switzerland and many other countries;
and a start has been made to integrate these programmes. These
three have been pioneers in this extended network which has
been given an international identity through the development of
the Association of Therapeutic Communities, and more recently
through the 'International Journal of Therapeutic Communities'
(Hinshelwood, 1980).

PROCESS

Process has become an increasingly important concept to me over
the years and is intimately linked with learning as a social process. In reaching our goal of an open system at Dingleton, we
came to realize that the process was more important than the goal
itself. When I was asked during my latter years at Dingleton

what I thought would be achieved in the next few years, I was unable to make a prediction; we were becoming much less goal-oriented, and were prepared to wait for things to 'happen'. This was in sharp contrast to the 'management by objectives', considered the efficient approach to planning popular at that time. In other words, we were learning about learning and came to realize that in the pursuit of knowledge, we might have missed the lessons of the process.

We were ready to change our goal orientation at any time if the circumstances seemed to indicate that our original plan had become inappropriate. Our original paradigm might be replaced by a new paradigm which, by implication, could itself be changed through time by new awareness or circumstance. This degree of flexibility reflects the uncertainty associated with a climate for change, which in turn shows how far we had moved from the scientific reductivism so characteristic of medical establishments. Change became associated with the process of learning and had an exciting and enriching quality very different from the more typical resistance to, and fear of, change.

INTUITION

This open-mindedness and willingness to change, together with uncertainty in terms of the extent and direction of our evolution, made intuitive thinking possible in addition to the more traditional reductive rational thinking. We felt free to challenge basic assumptions held by society at large. Social learning and growth include the concept of a paradigm shift - a paradigm being a temporary position in relation to an idea which may change at any time in the light of new information or in response to an intuitive feeling.

This willingness to change and acceptance of an intuitive aspect to process, learning and growth contributed to what my critics were pleased to call 'woolly' or illogical thinking. I no longer feared to admit ignorance or lack of proof, so-called 'hard data', in relation to many of our findings. This relates to the discussion of synthesis at the beginning of the chapter.

Brain research seems to indicate that the brain absorbs far more information than we are conscious of, and we only recognize what fits in with our expectations - the rest is disallowed from consciousness much as we ignore the 'blind spot', where the optic nerve breaks the continuity of the retina while the gap is filled in for us by the brain. It is now generally accepted that the two hemispheres of the brain serve different functions, though obviously interrelated. The left hemisphere represents our familiar self. It controls speech and is associated with our rational thinking. The right brain is associated with musical and artistic appreciation and abstract thinking. Without its involvement the left brain is less able to detect patterns and fill in gaps in our awareness from our past heritage - much like Carl Jung's

'universal unconscious'. Our traditional education is mainly limited to developing the left brain functions, largely excluding the right brain kind of activities. We prize reductive reasoning at the expense of our more artistic and creative potentialities. To achieve holistic thinking we need a balance of function between the two hemispheres. Without this integration we deny ourselves the development of our intuitive potential. The 'Concise Oxford Dictionary' defines intuition as 'immediate apprehension by the mind without reasoning'. I see this willingness to accept 'hunches' or intuitive feelings as an essential part of social learning. It can overlap with judgment, as in the case of our confrontation with the Regional Board in Edinburgh described in Chapter 3. Not only had we a cause worth fighting for, a plan to select nurse trainees after they had worked with us for about a year as activity assistants, but it also 'felt' right. In fact I can trace a thread of intuitive thinking from my schooldays, when I risked the wrath of my own school administration for challenging a more powerful school at rugby football convinced that we would win, to the various evolutionary stages of therapeutic community practice usually accompanied by an intuition that we were on the right course. Initially, as pioneers, we had no way of 'knowing' that our deviant orientation was sound. It 'felt' right and attracted staff who resonated to the same intuitive philosophy, which in turn was shared by the patients through contagion.

Another way of looking at this phenomenon is to postulate that the brain absorbs endless information but, because of our predominant patterns of thought, very little reaches our consciousness. Our attention is largely focused on the familiar and the socially acceptable and not on a wider synthesis. This computer-like potential of the mind is now being studied intensively by brain researchers greatly helped by the emergence of hologram pictures. This is not the place to discuss such work, but it would appear that there is a growing awareness that holographic theory may ultimately afford proof of a link between man's mind, the abstract, the intuitive, the mystical or Eastern thought.

I know that for me the early morning (I usually wake at 3.00 a.m.) is the time when new ideas are apt to surface. In the shower, in a state of sleepiness and of diffuse attention, occasional flashes of understanding (new ideas) can occur. Everyone probably has his/her periods of open-mindedness; it seems reasonable to encourage such phenomena. Conscious attempts to engage in abstract or mystical thought are now a commonplace, but I have not attempted to learn the techniques of yoga, transcendental meditation, etc., although I am interested and see no contradiction with systems theory.

RISK-TAKING

Another essential ingredient in social learning is the presence of a risk-taker - someone who has an innate capacity, perhaps acquired by living in a 'free' environment, which allows the person to question, interact spontaneously and without his own internal censorship (Jones, 1976a, p. 38). Throughout this book Reg Elliott was such a person. In the traditional hospital culture before my arrival, his spontaneity had created trouble for him on many occasions, especially with the authority structure - so much so that his career as a nurse was in jeopardy. When I left Dingleton seven years later he was number three in the nursing hierarchy and his contribution to our growth had been enormous. I am limiting this concept to individuals with a serious commitment to a specific goal or ideal. Reg had rebelled against the abuse of authority by the nursing hierarchy from the start and was expressing the feelings experienced by the majority of his peers. It seemed that he was prepared to lose his job if necessary, even though he was married and aware of his family responsibilities. This risk-taker role has two dimensions: it reflects the commitment of the individual at risk, and at the same time tests the integrity and commitment of the person in authority who is challenged. My initial 'tilt' with Reg at our first open meeting with about sixty staff present demonstrated in action that criticism was welcome. It allowed for interaction and the formulation of different views regarding the same problem. Here was an early example of a living-learning situation and the forerunner of our concept of social learning.

My experience with this approach has convinced me of its validity, and I try to welcome the challenge despite the hurt and embarrassment which usually accompany it. I say 'try to', as it is a learned response based on the conviction that the outcome usually amounts to social learning. But sometimes this is impossible and I have already discussed the advantage of multiple leadership when a leader is too emotionally involved to remain objective, thus requiring an alternate leader to assume the facilitator role.

SOCIAL ENVIRONMENT

This is the last of the dimensions of social learning which will be discussed and is perhaps the most important. The social environment of a hospital or other institution is subject to change in accordance with innumerable variables, whether planned or unplanned.

The important known environmental factors which contributed to Dingleton's favourable social climate for change and growth included a hospital which was open to the outside world - no locked wards, no front gate so that access to or from the adjacent small town of Melrose was unimpeded. Patients' visitors had

access to the hospital at any time of day, and had a delightful canteen where coffee and snacks could be enjoyed in a very comfortable environment - available to patients and staff alike. The architect, Peter Womersley, had reconstructed much of the building to give a pleasing and relaxed physical environment. The entrance hall was worthy of an exclusive club with comfortable armchairs and an enlarged photomural of the River Tweed covering the entire wall. Behind the reception window was a secretary whose function was partly to welcome visitors, answer questions, and find an appropriate staff member if that was called for. The high 'institutional' ceiling in the dining hall, shared by patients and staff, had been lowered and the large windows with colourful drapes looked on to the hospital grounds which, together with small individual tables and well-designed cafeteria, combined function with an aesthetic environment. Some of the geriatric wards were in the basement and originally had been dark and forbidding. The architect had removed the outside wall and these wards now had an uninterrupted view of a pleasant wood. The elderly men were allowed a 'nightcap' to encourage both social interaction and sleep.

It would become repetitious to enumerate the endless evidences of a social scene compatible with social interaction and which made Dingleton so distinctive. Add to these factors the formal organization of meetings available to all patients and staff where treatment and training overlapped and we have the beginning of an environment conducive to the process of change.

A therapeutic community is a deliberate attempt to synthesize a social structure which optimizes the opportunities for social learning, growth and creativity. That such a system, like all social systems, is in a constant state of flux is generally accepted, but an open system makes possible various checks and balances which tend to restore an equilibrium and, at the same time, avoid a static state of institutionalization. If growth is the process by which things become connected with each other and as a consequence come to operate at higher levels of organization and complexity, then not only were our connections (communications) within Dingleton as open as we could manage (feedback), but we were sensitive to our connections in the environment (feed forward). This latter helped to balance our internal social structure with the ever-changing scene outside the hospital, which in turn helped to limit distortion of information, rumour, etc.

The social environment at Dingleton changed in many ways during my stay there, as outlined in the preceding chapters. At first we inherited from my predecessor a fairly traditional hierarchical social structure with most administrative decisions unilaterally made by him. Within days of my arrival the beginnings of two-way communication, information-sharing and shared decision-making were instituted by the establishment of various meetings. By removing the controls from a central authority the hospital identity was changed almost overnight. Many more staff

had to share in the responsibility for the hospital - 'the' hospital
changed to 'our' hospital. Growth of a new value system and responsibility was rapid, but change brought confusion, too, and
depending on such variables as status and commitment to the
task, resistances to change and charges of exploitation, etc.,
grew. But the process of growth retained its momentum as more
and more variables were recognized, identified in connection with
the system as a whole, and if appropriate adopted. The infiltration
of the surrounding environment of the hospital widened the
system, and feedback as well as feed forward helped to form
links throughout the system and foster both equilibrium and
growth. At no time did we seem to be seriously out of tune with
our environment. On the other hand, our relationship with the
central authority in Edinburgh suffered by the absence of these
communication links - in both directions.

As already indicated at the beginning of this chapter I chose,
somewhat arbitrarily, twelve factors which were in some way
connected with the concept of social learning. These factors
might well be implemented by the addition of innumerable other
variables, many of which still elude identification, and even if,
in this context, the system was complete (impossible to conceptualize) the sum of the parts would not give the full meaning
of the whole - social learning.

Chapter 9

Epilogue: social learning, growth and creativity as process-products of open systems

Resistance to change is an inherent quality of man, consolidated in our Western culture with its emphasis on conformity, starting in the home and extending to schools, colleges and employment. Perhaps even more negative are our cultural values of power, money and 'success' at any cost. Most people who enter the 'rat race' fail in this struggle to reach 'the top' and lapse into a bored routine or even mental illness at one extreme, or take short cuts to 'success' by sacrificing moral values or by turning to crime at the other extreme. The by-products of this age of disillusionment include racial hatred, extreme poverty living beside affluence in an increasing atmosphere of tension, nationalism, isolationism and false hopes that technology alone will supply the answer to these problems.

The more insecure the world is, the greater the temptation to achieve 'security' through power, money and prestige, and so insulate ourselves from the 'mob'. Thus, the rich grow richer and the poor poorer. Even so, many of the lucky ones would seem to have an uneasy awareness that the present course of events may lead to disaster.

The perpetuation of such a value system is spawning its own reaction in the form of a growing explosiveness of the 'have nots' in the Third World. In this book we have discussed one model for change which, in its general outlines, has a universal application, and a message of hope. I am well aware that to argue from my very limited experience of systems theory and change as described in this book to systems in general on a large scale is to invite severe criticism. However, I believe that in the present state of world confusion the holistic approach advocated is fully justified.

My interest in open systems began as a vague awareness of the possibility of mobilizing the forces in the social environment to bring about change with groups of disadvantaged people. The process associated with these changes led to a preoccupation with social learning as described in the previous chapter. My growing interest in the process of change led me to realize that growth and creativity are, at least in part, a by-product of an open system. If we see social learning, growth and creativity as a continuum, then I would like to consider creativity in its place in the continuum. I believe that creativity is potentially present in everyone and not limited to the concept of genius or exceptional people. My wife is an artist and has helped me enormously to conceptualize the transition from social learning and open

systems to a more comprehensive view of creativity (C. Jones, 1978).

Before discussing creativity, it is important to reconsider some basic concepts about general systems theory. A system has a boundary that sets it apart from other things in its environment - it takes in things from its environment and puts other things out into the environment. A mature system is more than a sum of its parts. It is synergetic; that is, it can only be comprehended as 'product', where there is a compound effect when the parts interact with each other (Land and Kenneally, 1977, p. 15).

Whole systems must evolve and improve their ability to interconnect themselves internally, as well as with their environment. Any whole system not only has negative feedback (the self-regulation component of part systems in which errors are corrected, thus maintaining the status quo or 'homeostasis' - equilibrium); but it must also have positive feedback. Not only must it know what it has done wrong, but also what it has done right. It must not only have feedback, but it must have feed forward; that is, new information must be taken in from its environment in order to meet continuously the needs of properly connecting with a changing environment (Land and Kenneally, 1977, p. 18). This connecting phenomenon is 'growth'. Growth is the process by which things become connected with each other and operate at higher levels of organization and complexity.

As in the case of growth, there are levels of creativity, as when an idea or concept can no longer grow unless it links up with other viable concepts. The resulting creative product takes on the attributes of synergy - the whole is greater than the sum of the parts. Beyond this level is the need to explore other combinations and find a way to recombine the old concept at a higher level of relationship to the environment. For this step to occur there must be a 'destructuring' of what exists. One has to take a risk and become insecure and vulnerable to reach this stage of transformation. It involves a sort of 'loss of identity', where the person or organization or idea is breaking apart and there is a period of necessary exploration of a new unknown environment (a new disorder). It is only through this 'unknown' that a new order and a new combination or a new identity can be discovered. Koestler described this level (Flach, 1978, p. 109):

> the process of taking a step backward in order to take a leap forward as an integral part of the human experience of learning and change.
> . . . We found this pattern repeated on the level of human creativity; the scientist, faced by a perplexing situation must plunge into a 'dark night of the soul' before he can reemerge into the light. The history of the sciences and arts is a tale of recurrent crises, of traumatic challenges, which entail a temporary disintegration of the traditional forms of reasoning and perception and a new innocence of the eye; followed by

the liberation from restraint of creative potentials, and their reintegration into a new synthesis.

What does all this mean? Simply that there are different degrees, levels (of maturation, if you like) of creativity, of growth and of social systems. To say that 'this is true creativity and this is not' is looking at the part and not the whole system of development. In other words, creativity is relative to its creator as an individual and where he/she is in his/her level of growth; it is relative to the level of development of the social system or environment in which this creator lives; and it is relative to the whole system at the highest possible level of development thus far achieved.

If we look at the history of man and his accomplishments, we notice that creative people who reach the rank of genius appear in particularly large numbers in certain periods of history in given geographical areas. ('Genius' is used to describe a human being who has an extraordinary capacity for desirable originality, or who makes a new and profound contribution to some or all of mankind. In other words, an individual functioning at a very high level of growth, who lives in an environment of high development and maturity.) This uneven distribution suggests that special environmental circumstances are a determining factor in the occurrence of a high level of creativity. Take three major examples in history - the classic Greek period, the Italian Renaissance and the time of the American Revolution - they show that creativity does not occur at random, but is enhanced by environmental factors. In a systems perspective, what I am proposing is that there are many more individuals who possess the capacity for the highest level of growth and creativity than achieve it. There are also many others whose capacity may be less, but who are also living and functioning much below their potential. As Parnes states (1970, p. 352): 'Many people seem to possess the seeds of creativeness, but the social system or environment fails to provide the proper nourishment for growth.'

What is this environment or social system that nourishes and fosters growth and creativity? It would seem that it is an open social system operating at a high level of development or growth. We do much talking about the traits of a creative individual. I am suggesting that these traits of a creative individual are equally applicable to a creative open social environment. Chris Argyris defines an open system as follows (1970, p. 136):

An open system is one whose strategy for adaption is less on building defensive forts and more on reaching out, learning, and becoming competent in controlling the external and internal environment so that its objectives are achieved and its members continue to learn (and grow). An open system not only is open to being influenced, but also its members strive to accept every responsibility that helps them increase their

capacity to solve problems effectively.

Table 1 correlates the traits of a creative individual with those of a creative environment.

Table 1

Traits of a creative person	Traits of a creative environment
Sensitive - ability to see problems holistically - observant	Information-sharing, listening, interacting and learning as a social process; system is sensitive to problems through effective communication channels; works through problems as a group rather than ignoring them or solving them by administrative fiat.
Flexible - adaptive	Problem-solving facilitated by social structure; regularly scheduled meetings which set priorities as the group sees fit.
Spontaneous	Emergency meetings aided by flexible social system; no unnecessary delays; access to all members because of efficient communication channels.
Original - unusual responses - not tied to convention	There is no 'one' open system. Every truly open system has a unique identity dependent upon the individuals who constitute the system, and how far they realize their latent potential.
Ability to share	Much attention is paid to two-way communication of content and feeling, to sharing of information, and to shared decision-making.
Redefining - improvising - elaborating	Feed forward - new information taken in from its environment.
Interest in reflective thinking	Recycling - input, output, throughput, response to environment; always evaluating where it is at, how it is functioning, whether it is meeting needs.
Tolerance for conflicting information	Encourages all points of view and welcomes conflicting inputs.
Tolerance for ambiguity	Can 'table' and work through at a later date(s) important issues which come up and cannot yet be solved by consensus.

Table 1   (cont'd)

Traits of a creative person	Traits of a creative environment
Confident	Atmosphere of mutual trust and respect; belief in ability to solve problems; high degree of commitment and trust dependent on effective leadership.
Perceptive v. judgmental (is aware of various possibilities rather than coming to a conclusion about something)	Handles issues that come up with an 'open mind' - careful not to prejudge situations.
Openness to experience - lack of rigidity	Structure always evolving; not held to long-range goals and plans which the system must be a 'slave' to; it structures and restructures itself as needs arise.
Internal source of evaluation	Negative feedback and positive feedback; errors are corrected, but learning is the focus, not judgment; 'strokes' given for positive inputs, etc.; positive criticism is an essential part of growth.
Healthy scepticism	Does not accept status quo; always evaluating and changing as necessary; can laugh at oneself.
Sincere desire to help mankind	Positive social learning is the focus rather than determining who is wrong or finding blame.
Emotional, mental and physical drive	High morale and energy level.
Risk-taker; able to be insecure and vulnerable	Destructuring of what exists so that higher levels of reintegration are possible; there is enough confidence and trust in the system to take risks; secure from fear of reprisal.
Ability to use errors and to have a detached devotion - objectivity	Facilitator role in a social system - stays objective; does not judge; helps system to help itself. Positive criticism.
Unconventional thinking - nonconformist	Solutions arrived at may challenge social norms of the larger society.
Avoids suppression as a mechanism for control of conflicts; recognizes ego defences	Works through conflicts; invites confrontation and working through of these conflicts.

Table 1   (cont'd)

Traits of a creative person	Traits of a creative environment
More capable of holding and comparing many ideas; hence making a richer synthesis	Functions by finding consensus; thus, all viewpoints in the system attempt a synthesis.

In brief, a connection between open systems, growth and creativity is postulated – they form a continuum. Although it is generally accepted that to some extent everyone is the product of his/her environment, we suggest that growth and creativity are more easily conceptualized in connection with an open system. Heredity, adversity and many other factors are also important. However, our experience in a microcosm of society at Dingleton represented for many of us a new philosophy of life. A group identity in a supportive setting makes one not only less vulnerable but makes possible various dimensions of social learning, as was discussed in Chapter 8. This group identity within an open system contributes to positive living and is a protection against many of the social and political problems of our time. The dynamic challenging quality associated with an open system, its correlation with the biological systems found in nature, the feeling of fulfilment and high morale which is experienced by the people comprising the system, together with an awareness of a new capacity to learn and grow, all support my belief in this approach.

For me it has been a natural transition from open systems theory and practice, in a microcosm of society such as a hospital, to a consideration of the various aspects of a counterculture which, like so many others, I see evolving world-wide. It is as though our tiny stream of social reorganization and change starting in the mid-1940s has joined up with many tributaries from diverse areas of human endeavour to produce a large volume of material, which has been brilliantly summarized by Marilyn Ferguson (1981) who coined the term 'Aquarian conspiracy' (Aquarius, the water-bearer in the ancient zodiac – flowing water and quenching of thirst; conspiracy – an intimate joining). Like many other people she talks about the social activism of the 1960s and the consciousness revolution of the early 1970s, moving toward a synthesis of community action as a response to the abuse of power, money and privilege in our Western culture. This counterculture is evidenced by an amazing number of organizations and periodicals dedicated to a new and better world concerned with respecting and saving the environment and man himself. These are annotated in her book so that anyone may join the network of his/her choice, whether it be combating world hunger, counselling the terminally ill, a national

network of those interested in creativity, or an international organization offering a matrix of many networks and activities, conferences, bibliographies, lists of growth centres, educational programmes, etc. It has been said that as many as 15 million Americans belong to these networks. The BBC created a television series, 'Grapevine: The Self Help Show', to help people find suitable networks.

In this context of a counterculture one must mention a group of prominent writers, sometimes called 'Futurists' including such names as Alvin Toffler (1970), E.F. Schumacher (1974), Theodore Roszak (1978), William Irwin Thompson (1973), Ivan Illich (1971), Hazel Henderson (1978), Gregory Bateson (1972) and Arthur Koestler (1975).

It is impossible to condense the work of the eight 'Futurists' mentioned, but to some extent Marilyn Ferguson undertakes this formidable task. For her courage many purists may call her superficial, but to me she seems to embrace a vast area with considerable skill. Perhaps Hazel Henderson, by limiting herself largely to the socio-economic field, is on safer ground. Her basic attitude might be summed up in one sentence, 'We must now run our economy with a leaner mix of capital, energy and materials and a richer mix of labour and human resources' (1978, p. 7).

I was fortunate in having several meetings with Aldous Huxley, who was sufficiently interested in the concept of a therapeutic community to spend two days with us to study at first hand the therapeutic community at Oregon State Hospital in 1962. Arthur Koestler also showed a great interest in therapeutic communities and I spent many hours with him discussing this subject during the Second World War. Both these authors were preoccupied with the need to tap man's latent potential and thus enhance both growth and creativity.

From my reading and contacts in these and other fields I find a remarkable consonance with our concept of a therapeutic culture which has evolved over the past, almost forty, years. This, together with the growing body of knowledge in the human and biological sciences, largely endorses our findings in relation to the process of change, social learning, growth and creativity.

Bibliography

Argyris, C. (1970), 'Intervention Theory and Method', Reading,
Addison-Wesley.

Bateson, G. (1972), 'Steps to an Ecology of Mind', New York,
Ballantine Books.

Buckley, W. (1967), 'Sociology and Modern Systems Theory',
Englewood Cliffs, New Jersey, Prentice-Hall.

Caudill, W. (1958), 'The Psychiatric Hospital as a Small Society',
Boston, Mass., Harvard University Press.

Fairweather, G. et al. (1974), 'Creating Change in Mental Health
Organizations', New York, Pergamon Press.

Ferguson, M. (1981), 'The Aquarian Conspiracy', London,
Routledge & Kegan Paul.

Flach, F. (1978), A reappraisal of the creative process, 'Psychiatric Annals', March, vol. 8, p. 109.

Garcia, L.B. (1960), The Clarinda plan - an ecological approach
to hospital organization, 'Mental Hospital', November, pp. 30-1.

Henderson, H. (1978), 'Creating Alternative Futures', New York,
Berkley Publishing Co.

Hinshelwood, R.D. (ed), 'International Journal of Therapeutic
Communities', New York, Human Sciences Press, vol. 1, no. 1.

Illich, I. (1971), 'Deschooling Society', New York, Harper &
Row.

Jones, C. (1978), Creativity and the social environment, unpub-
lished paper.

Jones, M. (1948), Physiological and psychological responses to
stress in neurotic patients, 'Journal of Mental Science', vol.
44, no. 395, pp. 392-427.

Jones, M. (1952), 'Social Psychiatry: A Study of Therapeutic
Communities', London, Tavistock Publications; also published
in the USA in 1953 as 'The Therapeutic Community: A New
Treatment Method in Psychiatry', New York, Basic Books.

Jones, M. (1962), 'Social Psychiatry: in the Community, in
Hospitals, and in Prisons', Springfield, Ill., Charles C.
Thomas.

Jones, M. (1963), What is psychiatric nursing, 'Lancet', vol. 2,
pp. 1108-10.

Jones, M. (1964), Psychiatric nursing is out of tune in the USA,
'American Journal of Nursing', January, pp. 103-5.

Jones, M. (1968a), 'Beyond the Therapeutic Community: Social
Learning and Social Psychiatry', New Haven, Conn., Yale
University Press.

Jones, M. (1968b), 'Social Psychiatry in Practice', Harmonds-

worth, Middx, Penguin Books.

Jones, M. (1974), Psychiatry, systems theory, education, and change, 'British Journal of Psychiatry', vol. 124, no. 578, pp. 75-80.

Jones, M. (1976a), 'Maturation of the Therapeutic Community: An Organic Approach to Health and Mental Health', New York, Human Sciences Press.

Jones, M. (1976b), Using a facilitator as a change agent in social systems, 'Hospital and Community Psychiatry', March, vol. 27, no. 3, pp. 198-9.

Jones, M. (1979a), Social learning and social change, in R.D. Hinshelwood and N. Manning (eds), 'Therapeutic Communities: Reflections and Progress', London, Routledge & Kegan Paul, pp. 1-9.

Jones, M. (1979b), State mental hospitals and the future, 'Psychiatric Quarterly', vol. 51, no. 2, pp. 151-60.

Jones, M. (1979c), Therapeutic Communities old and new, 'American Journal of Drug and Alcohol Abuse', vol. 6, no. 2, pp. 137-49.

Jones, M. and Clark, M. (1965), Social psychiatry and the senior nurse, 'Nursing Mirror', 9 and 16 April, pp. 45-7 and 64-6.

Jones, M. and Dewer, J. (1964) Whither psychiatric nursing, 'Nursing Times', vol. 60, pp. 731-3.

Jones, M. and Mullen, C. (1963), What psychiatric nursing is about, 'Nursing Times, vol. 59, pp. 701-3.

Jones, M. and Polak, P. (1968), Crisis and confrontation, 'British Journal of Psychiatry', vol. 114, pp. 169-74.

Jones, M. and Stanford, G. (1973), Transforming schools into learning communities, 'Phi Delta Kappan', November, pp. 201, 203, 223-4.

Koestler, A. (1975), 'The Act of Creation', London, Picador.

Land, G. (1973), 'Grow or Die', New York, Delta Books.

Land, G. and Kenneally, C. (1977), Creativity, reality and general systems: a personal viewpoint, 'Journal of Creative Behavior', vol. 11, first quarter, pp. 12-35.

Lippit, P. and Lohman, J.E. (1965), Cross-age relationships, an educational resource, 'Children', vol. 12, pp. 113-17.

Martin, D. (1962), 'Adventure in Psychiatry', London, Faber & Faber.

Murrell, S.A. (1973), 'Community Psychology and Social Systems', New York, Behavioral Publications.

Parnes, S.J. (1970), Education and creativity, in P.E. Vernon (ed.), 'Creativity', Harmondsworth, Middx, Penguin Books, pp. 341-54.

Parsons, T. (1960), General theory in sociology, in R.K. Merton, L. Brown and L.S. Cottrell (eds), 'Sociology Today', New York, Basic Books, pp. 3-38.

Peele, R. et al. (1977), Asylums revisited, 'American Journal of Psychiatry', October, vol. 134, no. 10.

Roszak, T. (1978), 'Person/Planet', New York, Anchor Press-Doubleday.

Schumacher, E.F. (1974), 'Small is Beautiful', London, Sphere
  Books.
Scottish Home and Health Department (1968), 'Administrative Re-
  organization of the Scottish Health Services', Edinburgh, HMSO.
Stanton, A.H. and Swartz, M.S. (1954), 'The Mental Hospital',
  New York, Basic Books.
Stobie, E.G. and Hopkins, D. (1972), Crisis intervention 1:
  A psychiatric community nurse in a rural area, 'Nursing
  Times', 26 October, pp. 165-8; and Crisis intervention 2: A
  psychiatric community nurse in a rural area, 'Nursing Times',
  2 November, pp. 169-72.
Thompson, W.I. (1973), 'Passages About Earth', New York,
  Harper & Row.
Toffler, A. (1970), 'Future Shock', New York, Random House.
Tuxford, J. (1952), Follow-up inquiry I - Some general aspects,
  in M. Jones, 'Social Psychiatry: A Study of Therapeutic
  Communities', London, Tavistock Publications, pp. 96-106.
US President (1963), 'Message of the President of the US Relative
  to Mental Illness and Mental Retardation', Washington, D.C,
  88th Congress, First Session, House of Representatives,
  5 February, J.F. Kennedy, document no. 58.

Index